WHAT'S DRIVING DEMAND FOR DRUG USE IN THE UNITED STATE

A Forensic Qualitative Therapy Process Analysis for
Understanding, Treating and Preventing Relapse

GOOD FOR

COUNSELORS, CHURCHES, COLLEGES, MDS', FAMILIES, FRIENDS, LAW
ENFORCEMENT, ATTORNEYS OF MENTAL HEALTH COURTS, POLICY MAKERS,
PROGRAM MANAGERS, PSYCHOLOGISTS, SOCIAL WORKERS, SCHOOLS,
STUDENTS, THERAPIST AND UNIVERSITES

DR. RICHARD CORKER-CAULKER, PH. D. EDDCP

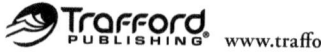 www.trafford.com

North America & international
toll-free: 1 888 232 4444 (USA & Canada)
fax: 812 355 4082

ABSTRACT

Review of the Findings

The author discovered he could adapt qualitative research methodology into a group therapy process for understanding pretreatment addiction relapse triggers. The author looked at many other therapy models and research models and decided on qualitative method as the viable possibility with good potential for identifying and understanding pretreatment addiction in a large group of over thirty individuals. The approach was successful at determining the varied relapse factors for individuals as well as more common relapse responses given by the group. As such, the approach can be used by clinicians facilitating such education, to provide a greater level of knowledge and understanding of the individual factors representing real risks for these group participants that need to be addressed for successful relapse prevention. Without addressing the predominant relapse triggers for these individuals, it becomes more likely that the relapse prevention will fail to be effective.

A review of the findings is presented according to the research questions of the study.

The results of the study from the data analysis demonstrate the multilevel effects of personal experience on personal relapse. External and internal factors were found and described by participants from the community and family level to an individual level. Relapse triggers were described by participants in terms of social and environmental factors, which, from the review of the literature, was somewhat expected. However, participants also noted individual, intrinsic factors, such as emotional states or problems that served to precipitate relapse, such as depression, sadness, aggression, anger, stress/anxiety, low self-esteem, and self-doubt. The study suggests the critical nature of addressing these psychological responses to drug use not only as a COD but also as a specific trigger for relapse.

According to the findings revealed from the data analysis, participants revealed a variety of causes for addiction relapse. The most common causes given by these group participants included social situations and social problems such as family problems and daily social situations and social relationships, including environmental triggers within the community of people, places, and things that call to mind using behaviors (peer pressure, or being around others who are still using); emotional problems such as anger, aggression, extreme sadness, or depression; and behaviors associated with a personal identification as an addict. Personal psychological triggers associated with self-doubt, low self-esteem, and stress and/or anxiety were also reported by participants often.

These perceptions also shed light on the nature of relapse specifically for this population. Although what would be considered to be typical relapse triggers according to the research, such as social situations/relationships, environmental, and community triggers, this population with COD also noted psychological factors of emotional problems, self-doubt, anxiety, and personal identification as an addict as additional or compounding addiction triggers.

According to the findings revealed in this study, providing assistance in developing strategies to handle social situations, relationships, and problems without relapsing would be beneficial to reducing the rate of relapse. Through the qualitative group approach, these strategies can be developed for very specific circumstances; for example, one participant noted a common trigger of food, due to the previous habit of taking LSD with food. A specific strategy can be developed for this individual in terms of finding an appropriate action plan for dealing with that specific trigger. Other triggers are more general and can incorporate the use of a more general, group-designed strategy, such as maintaining a support group to deal with social or emotional support issues that may arise.

It is noted, however, that within this population of individuals with COD, specific attention should be given to emotional/psychological responses to drug use and/or relapse. Counseling directed toward treatment processes for depression, mood disorders, general anxiety, or stress management, as well as issues of self-doubt and self-esteem, need to be added as a relapse prevention strategy. The personal identification of these individuals with drug use should also be addressed, perhaps through a focus on a reexamination of the individual and their personal strengths and weaknesses to develop a more concrete perception of self outside the realm of drug use.

Results from this study also underscore the importance of simultaneous treatment of the underlying co-occurring disorders and the reported psychological effects of drug use within this population, as psychological problems were noted not only as a cause for initial drug use and relapse but also as a personal trigger for these participants.

ACKNOWLEDGEMENTS

The author would like to acknowledge his fellow colleagues that worked with him in addiction treatment in private and public service, including the academic staff, drug court, hospitals, clinics, and jail setting—not forgetting his family, editors, typists, and all individuals that contributed to his awareness and understanding of the problem of pretreatment addiction relapse triggers and the need to develop knowledge, tools, skills, and analysis steps on the topic presented in this book. Finally, the author thanks the only wise God for his love and prosperity wishes for all.

DEDICATION

I would like to dedicate this book to all individuals affected by drug use and those struggling to overcome addiction—also to the many individuals we have lost in the struggle, not forgetting individuals with interest in the topic of addiction and all persons that will be inspired from reading this book and will dedicate time to serve individuals and families affected by pretreatment relapse triggers, problems, and challenges. I would also like to thank my wife and daughters for their support. Finally, I want to thank the one and only true God of creation that created us all in his image and likeness, with special abilities to subdue and govern the earth and its resources with promises of good health and prosperity for all.

TABLE OF TABLES

TABLE OF FIGURES

CONTENTS

CHAPTER ONE

Introduction

Relapse is common in drug and alcohol treatment. It is estimated that a good number of people trying to stay clean and sober have at least one relapse before they are able to stay clean and sober. But from experience, relapse or a "slip" does not begin on the day you relapsed or are arrested. It is a slow process. Some people say they had dreams they were using drugs before they relapsed, or they stop attending to or doing things that help them stay clean and then relapsed. Relapse behavior may be influenced by unknown pretreatment addiction relapse triggers. Therefore, the subject of pretreatment addiction relapse triggers demands a new examination for a better and more adequate understanding of pretreatment addiction relapse triggers all across our communities, where most crimes associated with drug and alcohol use occur and arrests are made before a person is sent to jail. Arrest and jail cannot be substitutes for the failure in developing therapy models and tools for identifying and analyzing underlying pretreatment addiction relapse triggers, thus forcing many to look for chemical control to escape. At the moment, therapy model and analysis tools needed to help clinicians, policy makers, and individuals and their families affected by drug use are lacking. Also, the problem gets more complicated if information about pretreatment addiction relapse triggers has not been compiled and made available to counselors and therapists working with forensic individuals within the criminal system. Psychotherapy model and analysis tools for identifying, processing, and analyzing the risks posed by pretreatment addiction relapse triggers is very important and urgently needed to plan interventions to prevent ongoing relapse or recidivism.

Drug and alcohol dependence is not a problem of those who produce, sell, buy, and use drugs but is a community problem because most relapse takes place in the community from where most people are arrested before they are sent to jail and referred to drug treatment for help. This makes it all the more relevant and important; no one will disagree, to develop a therapy model, analysis steps, and information on pretreatment addiction relapse triggers in the community as a contribution to improve understanding and developing effective treatment interventions for minimizing relapse.

It is not only families that will benefit from available information on pretreatment addiction relapse triggers, but clinicians, students, and community will also benefit if someone finds a way of how this can be done by compiling information on pretreatment addiction relapse triggers for understanding and planning treatment intervention.

As a clinician, the difficulty comes as one encounters individuals from different units on the case load of other therapists referred to your group for education for recovery in addiction treatment and you are compelled by sheer force of circumstances and numbers, from thirty-five to forty in a treatment group, to come up with tools for understanding the pretreatment addiction relapse triggers in the group than relying on general experience. Also, no two persons or groups are the same or will present the same pretreatment relapse triggers. Therefore, you have got to think out of the box immediately to come up with new models or tools that will help you learn about the pretreatment addiction triggers, find out the categories, patterns, and level of risk individuals will be exposed to. Developing a new therapy model is not easy to start because of cost, time, and commitment. It is a lot easier to keep using what is available than develop a new therapy model to capture, identify, and analyze pretreatment addiction relapse triggers for better understanding and treatment. You see, when you earn a living as an addiction therapist, you need to do more for your patients to improve their life and help prevent ongoing relapse or recidivism. You can do more if the information and tool is already available or compiled on the condition you are treating. But if it is not, you have to think of how to get it done to improve treatment outcomes through scientific means. How to study pretreatment addiction relapse triggers, patterns, categories, and risk levels for understanding volatility of sobriety is of key importance. As a clinician, having the knowledge and skills to adapt your psycho-educational group and therapy to an understanding and analysis of pretreatment addiction relapse triggers is one step that can be taken to help individuals understand the nature of addiction and the risk levels an individual may have been exposed to before treatment or will after discharge into the community. The author's core mission for writing about qualitative therapy and analysis steps is to bring the next generation of addiction therapy model, knowledge, skills, and scientific technique readily accessible for identifying pretreatment addiction relapse trigger, analysis, and risk level and benefit from a cutting-edge scientific approach. This study was designed to provide information on the best approach on the theory and practice of qualitative therapy and analysis for understanding pretreatment addiction relapse trigger patterns, categories, and risk levels, for minimizing relapse. We can minimize the possibility of repeated relapse if we have a therapy model that will allow for identification of pretreatment addiction relapse triggers and for analysis and determination of risk levels of pretreatment addiction relapse triggers. This report will be very beneficial to clinicians and treatment programs in the business of planning drug and alcohol treatment. Also, it will have great potential for identifying trigger risk levels through use of scientific qualitative analysis method and group practice.

The researcher wrote this book to share how qualitative therapy model and analysis process and steps have a pioneering lead for understanding, identifying, analyzing risk levels, and treating pretreatment addiction relapse triggers. This is the future and a less cost-effective way to go for a user-friendly approach in drug treatment in the twenty-first century. The author has studied a broad range of research methods, searching for best methods with a broad range of potential and possibilities for identifying and analyzing pretreatment addiction relapse triggers and their risk levels. The author discovered that qualitative research method can be adapted into therapy model for identifying and analysis of pretreatment addiction relapse triggers without much risk to patients. It is also a scientific approach with a lot of promise in drug and alcohol treatment. There is a lot of reason to be more excited about the possibilities once we learn about the process and rule out potential risks from benefits in helping us understand pretreatment addiction relapse triggers: what they are, how they affect and trigger repeated relapse risk, and what can be done to help patients stay clean and sober.

One thing you should know is that pretreatment relapse triggers and lifestyle is shrouded in secrecy that enhances relapse behavior and often passes by unnoticed in treatment if tools are not available to identify the triggers, patterns, categories, and level of risk to individuals before they are released or have completed their treatment. Finding a tool that will help clinicians enhance practice in drug and alcohol treatment is, without question, urgent. Because, according to Young, Joe, Hassin, and St. Clair (2001), in the general population, the rate of recidivism or drug relapse is 86% two years after treatment, with the majority of the relapses occurring within six months of treatment. Relapse challenges leave many families and individuals affected by drug and alcohol and prescription medication overdose asking a lot of questions about what is driving relapse behavior if and when a friend or family has got hooked on drugs and alcohol beyond an occasional use or socially accepted occasion.

The topic of alcohol and drug abuse has been making news headlines around the world and in the United States. In the United States, attention on drug use continues to increase as more and more people are arrested under the influence or die of prescription drugs overdose. The problem of drug addiction and repeated relapse behavior occurs every day. Repeated relapse is affecting the life of addicts, their families, and community that spend tax dollars to respond. What is driving or influencing the behavior of drug use? What are the impacts of chemical addiction? What can you do to help? This book was written to answer these questions. The problem of addiction is real. It is not a fiction of any sort as some may want to pretend it is or pretend it has nothing to do with them.

Potential for relapse is always high when clients or individuals are released into the very community where they relapsed or were arrested from without having spent adequate time in treatment to process and reconstruct their pretreatment relapse life and triggers and using the information to construct a clean and sober life. While general information may be available on addiction, the absence of data on pretreatment relapse triggers affecting forensic population makes it a lot harder to plan specific treatment goals and objectives for reducing or minimizing relapse behavior in the community and constructing with a client a clean and sober life goals and objectives. Therefore, therapy is generally focused on the existing models that are partially focused on thoughts, feelings, and behavior modification.

According to Young et al. (2001), in the general population, the rate of recidivism is 86% two years after treatment, with the majority of the relapses occurring within six months of treatment. The problem of illegal drug use and repeated relapse is not only affecting the addicts but a whole community. Drug addiction and repeated relapse behavior before and after treatment has come to the attention of many local and state government officials and treatment program leaders in the United States. As new recruits join ranks of drug use, drug crime, possession, and arrest will continue to climb because of new users and new addicts getting addicted to street drugs and alcohol. This is not a young-people issue only because adults are equally addicted to drug use for performance enhancement or for fitting into the social circle. One thing is important to understand that triggers in the community will continue to present a big challenge to users and treatment specialists, including law enforcement. But right now, obvious triggers in the environment are playing a role, but information on pretreatment addiction triggers and how to identify and analyze pretreatment addiction relapse triggers may be lacking in many communities across the country. We need this information to devise a relapse prevention treatment before an individual is released into the same community where he or she relapsed and was arrested from. The absence of information on pretreatment relapse triggers makes developing treatment plans difficult not only for clinicians but also for law enforcement staff and drug courts' personnel directly involved with legal enforcement and commitment. From personal experience, the absence of information in print on pretreatment relapse triggers makes planning and coordinating discharge readiness and relapse prevention a lot difficult, especially when working with a large group in a forensic setting including jails, prison, drug court treatment, and other programs like behavioral health clinics and hospitals. The need or availability of information in print, describing pretreatment addiction relapse triggers, will be beneficial to clinicians for understanding pretreatment relapse addiction phase and lifestyle (Patton, 2002).

Young et al. (2001) above states, in the general population, the rate of recidivism is 86% two years after treatment, with the majority of the relapses occurring within six months of treatment.

While this is true, people will continue to hold different opinions about why this or that person is using and cannot stop or grow up and leave drugs and alcohol alone. Others will have different world views and beliefs about why people use drugs and cannot stop, and some may link drug use to legal, moral, or spiritual problems, which is why it is important to explain what exactly is going on with people battling with the disease of drug use. It is essential that we have an open mind and a broader view than a limited one. This cannot be done until we find a way of how to identify and analyze pretreatment addiction relapse triggers.

Therefore, the need for analysis of pretreatment addiction relapse triggers from the experience of a therapist's observation and years of experience cannot be overemphasized, as demand for this information is well overdue to clarify what exactly is addiction relapse trigger and why it is a stumbling block and barrier to sobriety for many. Until we find ways and means, people are not going to stop looking at it from their own perspective before analyzing. We should never forget that a family visiting their loved ones may hold a metaphysical explanation less scientific because they attribute bad behavior, drinking, or using drugs to some weird forces or unseen forces at work controlling their loved ones. Though strange, there are individuals who still believe in unseen forces or spiritual forces at work and responsible for influencing human behaviors. What are the modern theories of behavior? The first is called the psychodynamic theory that states man is driven by instinct present at birth: by Id or life, death, and sex. Ego is a reality check that evaluates when or whether to wait, and superego is a value check that always determines if it the best thing to do to preserve life and satisfy personal desires. The second is the humanistic theory that suggests people are driven by a certain kind of anxiety, need for freedom, and option in a world that has no meaning. Third, is the Adlerian theory that says behavior is driven by faulty notions and assumptions. Fourth is the theory of object relations, according to which behavior is driven by trying to integrate or relate to objects in their surrounding objects, meaning parents, friends, or people. Fifth is the Jung theory developed around the idea that people are driven not by instinct as Freud claimed but by social problems and the anxiety around the problem.

But what is driving people to use drugs in America? This is exactly what this book is about: learning about what is driving people to use street drugs in America and how you can help. Qualitative therapy process offers the best possibility of finding out reasons for addiction. Why is qualitative therapy and data analysis important in addiction treatment? Think of it this way: addiction treatment is about helping, supporting, and creating an environment for a person using drugs to stop and prevent ongoing or future use and relapse. To do this, we must find a way of learning about the disease not from what we already know from textbook but learning about the disease from the people affected by it and from the staff or clinicians working with the problem.

Also, when it comes to behavior problems like relapse and drug use, you really do not want to rely heavily on what you already know. You need new and ongoing data to help you conceptualize factors contributing to the relapse behavior from different people groups. Likewise, clinicians' exposure and day-to-day understanding about a specific disease process will be different. This takes us to the next big topic in this study of addiction disease with regard to human horizontal relationships and triggers. What we should understand is how the disease manifests itself in various areas of life: the social, economic, and political. Areas of life are very important contexts for understanding addiction disease and for identifying and categorizing pre-treatment relapse triggers.

Large amount of data is sitting in shelves and curriculum notes about a specific disease, which, if and when analyzed, can help provide a comprehensive understanding of the disease of addiction. Depending on how notes are used, they may hold a key for unlocking the present secret of a disease. Qualitative analytic treatment is the way to go if we are to respond to the disease of addiction including all diseases. A single addict and clinician may not have all the information for understanding the comprehensive nature of a disease but may have a piece; if put together and analyzed, it can give the new insight for the development of treatment of horizontal triggers of a disease.

This is where data analysis comes in handy. To analyze will require a team of analysts trained in the science of data analysis first to gather the data from notes and experience of group, individuals, and treating clinician/s about their general experience treating a disease. Analysts will then assemble the general information for analysis. Addiction data analysis is critical for the comprehensive understanding of addiction within a group and specific population.

This study was designed to describe qualitative therapy group model and qualitative analysis steps. In this book, the author describes the theory of qualitative therapy model and analysis steps. In chapter one and two, there is an introduction to qualitative therapy issues and theories. In chapter three, you will learn how to relate key qualitative or Q therapy concepts, principles, techniques, and strategies in group process for reconstructing pretreatment relapse triggers and for constructing a clean and sober life using an understanding of the client's perception. Also, in chapter four, you will learn how the author used qualitative analysis technique steps to analyze data. In chapter five, the author identified categories and triggers patterns on the chemical effect of drugs.

Background of the Problem

The problem of pretreatment relapse triggers is experienced by many addicts arrested, sent to jail with reference to a divergent treatment program to seek sobriety treatment before release or the next court appearance. Crime relating to drug use and under the influence of drugs will not stop. The rise in gun-related crimes against a person in the community, whether these crimes are drug, alcohol, mental illness related, or pure violence or anger, requires new understanding of triggers in the community where most crimes occur before a person relapses or acts out for whatever reason ascertained or not. What is disturbing is that information on pretreatment addiction triggers affecting forensic individuals is not readily available for planning treatment specific to their situation and challenges. Also, existing therapy model and analysis approach has not been developed for understanding pretreatment addiction relapse triggers. With these problems of tools and information, the way out is that someone has to take the time to think of a therapeutic tool or model scientific enough to allow identification and analysis. While general information may be available on addiction, the absence of data on pretreatment relapse triggers affecting forensic population makes it a lot harder to plan specific treatment goals and objectives for reducing or minimizing relapse behavior in the community. The present models for therapy, however effective they have been, were not developed to process and analyze pretreatment addiction relapse triggers. Therapy is generally focused on working with issues from cognitive, behavioral, emotive issues and challenges and reward for good behavior than to identify and analyze pretreatment addiction relapse triggers. The justification for developing a new therapy model, as in this case, qualitative therapy and qualitative therapy analysis for use in pretreatment addiction relapse screening, analysis, and treatment cannot be allowed to pass by unnoticed or overemphasized because we need the tool and information to plan an effective treatment based on scientific trigger analysis result and approach that is presently lacking in drug and alcohol treatment. The new treatment model should help with identification screening, analysis, and trigger risk assessment before planning intervention. You want to base treatment goals and objectives on scientific trigger risk analysis than anything else. Also, with trigger analyses, you should be able to develop more in-depth understanding of pretreatment addiction relapse trigger beyond speculation to better understanding about what is driving or what social forces are driving or pushing individuals to drug use and dependence. Analysis will provide insight on the chemical effect of drug on specific population or group. Qualitative therapy analysis will help you understand the impact of street drug chemicals on individuals to make a determination for further medical assessment referral. This is why developing a new therapy model and analysis steps like qualitative therapy is so important to get it done.

The truth is that at no time will an addict stop shopping for drugs or change his drug-seeking behavior. Street drugs and alcohol have a devastating impact on the addict, and finding ways of understanding specific triggers leading to drug-seeking behavior before an addict sets in motion the ways and means of accessing the drugs will be one positive way of helping an individual deal with triggers associated with a relapse. If the way or an approach to do this is not available, including information on pretreatment addiction relapse trigger, we stand a chance of not winning the fight to keep people sober and clean. Chemical in any drugs has a way of affecting systems, organs, body parts and functions. Information on how chemical addiction affects perception, understanding, feelings, judgment, determination, knowing, thinking, reason, logic, moral judgment, reflection, sentiment, disposition, imagination, notion, intent, and ideas will be useful to know once we develop the therapeutic model and analysis to find out how individuals are affected, what parts of the body and what drug is involved. Therefore, it is essential for any relapse prevention treatment method to respond to individual feelings, triggers, and stressors (Kelly, Gaither, & King, 2007) that may be driving the demand for more drug use to stabilize their mood or feelings before or after an event, etc. There is documented evidence that overstimulation of the body with mood-altering drugs over a period may lead to possible mental challenges or co-occurring disorders.

According to research, positive treatment results for individuals with co-occurring disorders (COD) such as mental illness and substance abuse are best achieved through the integration of screening, assessment, and treatment planning, addressing both the substance abuse and the mental illness within a shared context (Center for Substance Abuse Treatment [CSAT], 2005, 2007) may be helpful because COD can be complex. This integrated process requires a great deal of flexibility in terms of clinician skills and creativity to produce an effective treatment plan. Research has provided evidence for poor treatment outcomes in individuals with COD and the need for targeted treatment for the prevention of relapse (CSAT, 2005, 2007).

Everitt and Robbins (2005) suggested:

> Drug addiction is increasingly viewed as the endpoint of a series of transitions from initial drug use—when a drug is voluntarily taken because it has reinforcing, often hedonic, effects—through loss of control over this behavior, such that it becomes habitual and ultimately compulsive. (p. 1481)

According to the literature, the human brain manifests a relationship between addiction and addiction triggers through the ability to learn to anticipate reactions to stimuli (Pate, 2009), similar to Pavlov's classical conditioning paradigm (Carroll, 1998). As such, individuals may experience overwhelming memories and emotions associated with specific music to which they used to get high, or with a specific location where they used to buy the target drug of their addiction (e.g., drugs) (Jaffe, 2010). Pretreatment addiction relapse trigger can be any person, place, thing, or situation that reminds a person of drug or alcohol use (Urell, 2010). Common triggers include being around people with whom one previously used drugs, having money, getting paid, drinking, being involved in a social situation, and experiencing certain affective states such as anxiety, depression, or joy (Carroll, 1998).

The part of the brain affected by environmental triggers has been identified as the amygdala (see Figure 1). The amygdala is a small, almond-shaped structure located in the temporal lobes of the brain near the hippocampus. It is believed to be linked to individual emotions, behavior, and aggression, and controls fear responses, secretion of hormones, arousal, and the formulation of emotional memories (Cherry, n.d.). The lateral section of the amygdala receives inputs from the visual, auditory, somatosensory, and pain systems. The medial nucleus of the amygdala is connected to the olfactory system. The central nucleus connects with brainstem areas that control the expression of innate behavior associated with physiological responses (Le Doux, 2008). Most of the inputs to the amygdala involve exciting pathways that use glutamate as a transmitter system. Thus, epinephrine, dopamine, serotonin, and acetylcholine are released in the amygdala, which is responsible for influencing how excitatory and inhibitory neurons interact (Le Doux, 2008).

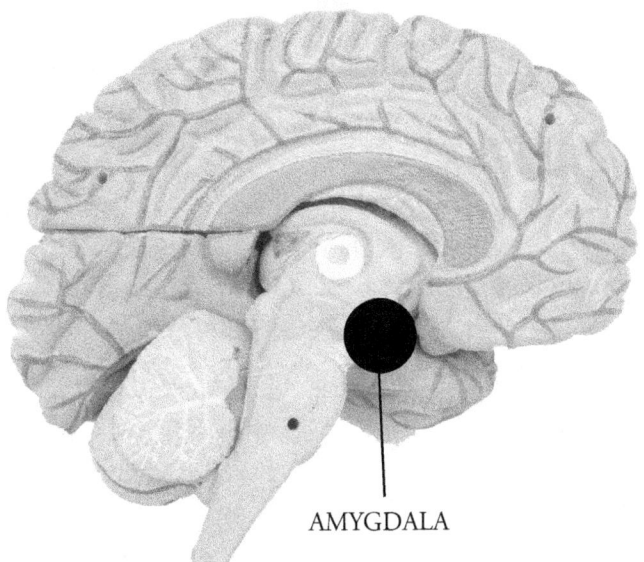

AMYGDALA

Figure 1. The human brain and position of the amygdala (*Source:* Thinkstockphotos.com).

The study by Le Doux (2008), sponsored by the National Institute of Drug Abuse, investigated the relationship between the amygdala and adjoining structures of the human brain. The researchers investigated the impact of dopamine on rats' behavior, including the brain receptors. Dopamine is a chemical messenger associated with pleasure and movement. The study identified the relationship between triggers and dopamine release in rats. The study first determined whether the amygdala plays a role in the effects of drug-use behavior. The researchers used rats trained to self-administer cocaine. According to the study, when the researcher inactivated the dopamine components in the areas of the extended amygdala in the rats, the rats significantly reduced the amount of cocaine they gave themselves. Reversely, if the dopamine component in the areas of the extended amygdala in rats is activated by a trigger, the resulting high levels of dopamine overstimulation will cause the number of dopamine receptors (i.e., the molecules to which the dopamine binds) to increase, causing the cocaine "high." This process accounts for cocaine addiction effects (Le Doux, 2008).

Statement of the Problem

What is clear is that from the study of the rats, we are able to understand the role that the brain plays and how it influences drug-seeking behavior and use. We know this because we have compiled information. If we are able to compile a study that will look at the analysis of pretreatment addiction relapse triggers, we would have accomplished a lot, particularly if the study showed how we could use new psychotherapy model to process and analyze pretreatment addiction relapse trigger and its risk levels to individuals that would eventually be discharged into the community and have to encounter relapse triggers. We can at least be able to use the information to inform our understanding with scientific process to support our delivery of care and any relevant intervention to minimize relapse or repeated recidivism before an individual is arrested for possession, use, or any other crime when under the influence. That is why the author is counting on this study to show how we can get this done, the study being cost-effective and scientific at the same time. Relapse prevention programs and drug and alcohol program in order to be effective must be targeted to specific triggers and stressors of individuals (Kelly et al., 2007). The gap in the literature on pretreatment relapse triggers among forensic individuals makes planning relapse prevention more difficult because information to start planning intervention targeting pretreatment relapse trigger may not be readily available for use until this study is completed and the information becomes available on pretreatment addiction relapse trigger qualitative group model and analysis steps.

Purpose of the Study

The reason this book was written was threefold: first, to describe how the author discovered and developed qualitative therapy and its application and use in education for recovery in addiction; secondly, how the author used qualitative analysis steps for identifying pretreatment addiction relapse trigger categories, patterns and risk levels; and thirdly, compile the information in one book for use by professionals when identifying, processing, and analyzing trigger categories, patterns, and risk levels before planning drug and alcohol treatment goals and objectives.

Conceptual Framework

The conceptual framework developed by the researcher for this study is drug and alcohol intervention should include a qualitative process and analysis of pretreatment addiction relapse trigger for understanding trigger risk levels and management of triggers to prevent relapse behavior and focus on abstinence, social, coping skills, non-social addictive behavior, a healthy and productive life (Beck, 1993; Kelly et al., 2007; Miller & Rollnick, 2009). Addiction treatment must resonate with general understanding of identified addiction relapse behavior associated with specific triggers and stressors that are often individualized and require identification to be successful in order to prevent or minimize repeated relapses (Kelly et al., 2007). Identification and analysis through use of qualitative analysis should take center stage in drug and alcohol treatment outcome alongside cognitive behavior therapy or CBT. Engaging in CBT without evidence of identification and analyses of an individual trigger or group may not prove very effective in the delivery of trigger reduction. Therefore, planning treatment without adequate identification and analysis of triggers is not a very effective approach, let alone relying and depending on general understanding of non-specific triggers to plan treatment. Therefore, adequate group therapy model for trigger identification, process, and analysis is important. There are existing psychotherapy models but not specifically designed for what we are talking about, a model that is designed and developed scientifically for identifying, processing, and exploring how pretreatment addiction relapse trigger risk poses serious challenge to sobriety. Pretreatment addiction trigger identification, analysis, risk, and resistance knowledge and skill training should be a major part of drug and alcohol treatment alongside cognitive behavior therapy. This is what qualitative therapy and analysis offer for present and future drug treatment. It is not about whether you want to develop a new therapy, but it is about a therapy model and analysis that offers the greatest possibilities for identifying, analyzing pretreatment addiction relapse triggers with resistance training for preventing repeated relapse. This is a fairly new approach but better late than never. The author will now comment on the existing models in the market.

Several psychotherapy models and methods have been in the public for some time. Therapists, including myself, use these methods to guide or plan the treatment of substance abuse or drug and alcohol. They include present use of cognitive behavior-behavioral therapy or CBT, motivational interviewing, and acceptance-based coping intervention (Kelly et al., 2007; Vieten, Astin, Buscemi, & Galloway, 2010). The goals of these treatment approaches are to focus the treatment on changing behavior (see Figure 2).

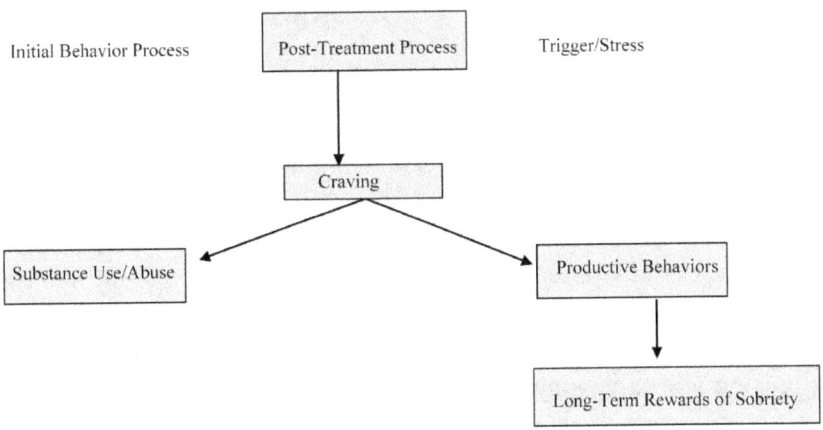

Figure 2. Behavioral therapy goal outline (adapted from Kelly et al., 2007).

Research Questions

The following research questions served to guide the author in analyzing the information on trigger and in writing the book. According to the data used in the analyses:

1. What will the data tell the author/researcher about the nature of addiction trigger among forensic population?
2. What are the causes, patterns, and categories of pretreatment addiction relapse triggers experienced by forensic individuals found in the data proposed for analysis?
3. Based on the study, what is the most effective way of treating pretreatment addiction relapse triggers?
4. How does qualitative group therapy approach in Education for Recovery in Addiction, which targets the revealed risks and pretreatment relapse triggers that contribute to the current research understanding of pretreatment addiction relapse prevention and discharge readiness before a client is released or discharged into the same community from where he or she relapsed and was arrested.

Limitations and Delimitations

The study is limited to pretreatment addiction relapse triggers. It is drawn from the author's observation, recollection, and data information on the topic analyzed in this study for writing this book. The information presented cannot be generalized beyond the topic, and it a presentation from the author's analysis result about development of qualitative therapy model and analysis for understanding and treating pretreatment addiction relapse triggers and their patterns, categories, and risk levels. While qualitative therapy models and practice present a promising scientific analysis approach in drug and alcohol treatment, it is not a solution to all problems because it is limited to group process and analysis for understanding pretreatment addiction relapse triggers in a more vivid representation, which otherwise would hardly have been possible without the therapy and analysis used in writing this book.

Definition of Terms

Terms used in the study analysis of the data are worth explaining because terms have different meanings in different contexts. Therefore, for the purposes of clarity, definitions of key terms used in the analysis have been provided. These are not necessarily universally accepted definitions.

Forensic Individuals: They are individuals admitted from the judicial system into treatment. They are identified by a commitment code such as court commitments, parole commitments, prison transfers, and civil commitments.

Pretreatment: This is a situation or condition before an individual starts receiving prescribed addiction treatment, including medication or individual or group therapy.

Addiction Treatment: It is a broad range of service for prescribed treatments. The overall goal of treatment is to reduce or eliminate drug use and restore an addict to productive life (Madigan, 2010).

Triggers: These include people, places, and things that contribute to a relapse, including thoughts, a craving to use, which are the most powerful triggers (US Department of Health and Human

Services [USHHS], 2009). Drug and alcohol triggers vary and are subjective from individual and social environment. This is why we cannot overemphasize to use the scientific approach developed in this study to first identify them and analyze them before treatment intervention is developed. They may include individual environment and socioeconomic challenges and other related problems like mental challenges, holiday, weekends, stress, or certain kinds of jobs that provide subjective defense for using or have come to associate with the need to use drugs and alcohol.

Addiction: It is a brain disease. It encompasses seeking and using drugs and alcohol, despite harmful consequences (National Institute on Drug Abuse [NIDA], 2010). Being addicted means giving up conscious control. Addiction is a progressive disease that causes impulsive and unconscious behavior (Dean, 2009).

Qualitative Method: It is a method of research that seeks to explore a phenomenon or problem by first trying to understand the problem from the perspective of the party, participant, individual, or the group studied. The goal is to try to get as much information as possible about the cause, nature, pattern, and category of the phenomenon or problem through the use of interviews, open questions and answers (Moustakas, 1995), personal observation, and notes documentation on the topic. Techniques employed in the process may include: (a) defining the problem; (b) developing the questions to ask in group process or analysis; (c) find individual, group, or data you want to use in your process or analysis; (d) develop a list of open questions about the phenomena about which you want to obtain information; (e) record, type, or write the answers down; and (f) store the information for analysis. The end product of qualitative research is a description of the phenomenon, including the data and how it was gathered and analyzed (Moustakas, 1995).

Qualitative Therapy: It is a psychosocial group developed by the author for use in Education for Recovery in Addiction. The author developed qualitative therapy in 2007. The author used qualitative research method in developing the therapy for exploring and processing the experiences of individuals with pretreatment addiction triggers and relapse problems. The researcher developed qualitative therapy with the assumption that individuals can be best treated in Education for Recovery in Addiction group, utilizing qualitative process.

The author developed qualitative therapy by applying the method of qualitative research process in education for recovery in addiction relapse prevention as follows: (a) identify the problem; (b) develop the questions to ask the group; (c) write down the answers given; (d) type the answers; (e) store the answers for group review and processing; and (f) use the information to develop a descriptive understanding of the problem and plan intervention with the group while respecting the contribution of the group or individual toward understanding the problem (Moustakas, 1995).

Data Population: This is an account of the population reflected in the topic notes used for group weekly follow-up and in the research analysis, generally including male and female individuals with some history of arrest and drug addiction that represents different ethnic groups and social class.

Data: The data used in the analysis did not include personal identifying information (names, addresses, date of birth, telephone numbers, e-mail addresses, Social Security numbers, voiceprints, fingerprints, photos, codes, diagnoses, or any other identifying characteristics). The notes used include anonymous data on the topic of pretreatment relapse triggers. The notes represent a diversity of general views and responses on pretreatment relapse triggers. Specifically, the notes included: (a) running accounts of diverse reflection and observation by the author; (b) theoretical information that included emergent trends; (c) hypotheses, which would have to be tested; (d) guesses and hunches; and (e) methodology notes on the process (Ratcliff, n.d.) used in the analysis.

Significance of the Study

The significance of learning about pretreatment addiction relapse triggers cannot be overemphasized, given the lack of resources on the topic specific to forensic population and the need to compile a data on the topic that can be used for group process and for understanding categories, patterns, and risks associated with pretreatment addiction relapse triggers and for preventing frequent relapse or other behavior problems associated with alcohol and drug use. Also, the need to develop and present a therapy model for group process and analysis of pretreatment addiction relapse triggers cannot be overemphasized as demand for understanding, identifying, and preventing the risk of pretreatment addiction relapse trigger continues. This risk has been documented by the United States White House of National Office of National Drug Control below.

The White House office of National Drug Control gives a descriptive picture of the reality of drug use in the United States as follows:

In 2007, the latest year for which data are available, 38,371 people died of drug-induced causes. The number of drug-induced deaths has grown from 19,128 in 1999, or from 6.8 deaths per 100,000 population to 12.6 in 2007.1 (These include causes directly involving drugs, such as accidental poisoning or overdoses, but do not include accidents, homicides, AIDS, and other causes indirectly related to drugs.)

There is a drug-induced death in the US every fifteen minutes. Compared to other causes of preventable deaths, drug-induced causes exceeded the 31,224 deaths from injuries due to firearms and the 23,199 alcohol-induced deaths recorded in 2007. In the same year, 34,598 deaths were classified as suicides and 18,361 deaths as homicides. From a national roadside survey in 2007, one in eight (12.4%) of weekend nighttime drivers tested positive for at least one illicit drug.

Based on a self-report survey in 2009, approximately 10.5 million Americans reported driving under the influence of an illicit drug during the past year. In 2009, one in three drivers killed in motor vehicle crashes, who were tested for drugs and the results known, tested positive for at least one medication or illicit drug. Among high school seniors in 2008, one in ten (10.4%) reported that in the two weeks prior to their interview, they had driven a vehicle after smoking marijuana.

The economic cost of drug abuse in the US was estimated at $180.9 billion in 2002, the last available estimate. This value represents both the use of resources to address health and crime consequences as well as the loss of potential productivity from disability, premature death, and withdrawal from the legitimate workforce.

In 2008, an estimated two million visits to emergency departments in US hospitals were associated with drug misuse or abuse, including close to one million (993,379) visits involving an illicit drug. Nonmedical use of pharmaceuticals was involved in 971,914 visits.

Cocaine was involved in 482,188 visits, marijuana was involved in 374,435 visits, heroin was involved in 200,666 visits, and stimulants (including amphetamines and methamphetamine) were involved in 91,939 visits.

According to a 2009 study of arrestees in ten major metropolitan areas across the country, drug use among the arrestee population is much higher than in the general US population. The percentage of booked arrestees testing positive for at least one illicit drug ranged from 56% to 82%. The most common substances present during tests, in descending order, are marijuana, cocaine, opiates (primarily metabolites of heroin or morphine), and methamphetamine. Many arrestees tested positive for more than one illegal drug at the time of arrest.

According to a 2004 survey of inmates in correctional facilities, 32% of state inmates and 26% of federal prisoners reported that they used drugs at the time of the offense. Addicts' potential for criminal behavior when under the influence may be very high (Office of National Drug Community Policy Executive office of the President, 2010). Pretreatment addiction triggers are experienced by many addicts. What is disturbing is we have less information if any at all on relapse caused due to pretreatment relapse triggers. Notes on pretreatment relapse triggers may have useful information for understanding the problem of pretreatment relapse triggers when analyzed and can be very useful as reference for learning about how to identify, analyze, and describe what pretreatment relapse triggers are for minimizing relapse.

The subject of pretreatment addiction relapse triggers plays a major role in relapse behavior. Therefore, the author takes the view that a more direct and effective way to treat addicts is to identify specific triggers, analyze the trigger, and learn about its categories, patterns, and risks before developing treatment to minimize its impact. The ongoing implication as we learn more about pretreatment addiction relapse triggers is what treatment we develop from the information. Keep in mind that the main concern of the author in writing this book is how to use the information on pretreatment addiction relapse triggers presented in the book in identifying, analyzing, understanding, and developing a treatment for minimizing triggers. The book is not about describing triggers but about how to identify, analyze, and study the dynamics of drug and alcohol triggers, including the chemical nature and effect of drugs on individuals.

An important contribution of the author is the effective use of qualitative or Q therapy for identifying, analyzing, and understanding pretreatment relapse triggers. The author contributed knowledge to the science of addiction and pretreatment relapse triggers by analyzing information on pretreatment relapse triggers. Triggers and stressors are generally specific (Kelly et al., 2007), therefore the author sought to describe and assess the efficacy of the use and application of qualitative therapy in alcohol and drug treatment, an approach new to drug treatment but effective for learning and understanding pretreatment relapse triggers and relapse prevention. It is obvious that the use of qualitative therapy will require training. The good thing about qualitative therapy from the author's experience as a therapist is that qualitative therapy practice in treatment groups is not complicated as one may be tempted to think. From the author's experience, the use of qualitative therapy in group therapy may require training for understanding the process and how it works. Equally important is the analyses of the therapist's reflection, comments, illustrations, questions, and ideas in understanding pretreatment relapse triggers. Analyses take time, and a therapist must be familiar with the process. A therapist can limit himself to just the use of qualitative therapy process group without going into analyses for more in-depth understanding of a problem. In this book, the author has presented both the description of how to conduct qualitative group therapy and how to analyze for understanding the dynamics of addiction triggers. A therapist is not under any obligation to do both. But doing both is fun and interesting. What do we know about triggers from the literature?

CHAPTER TWO

Literature Review

You are now in the literature review section of this book. As you progress, you are going to need this information to compare and contrast the analysis result presented in chapter four. Read and review the information in this chapter on triggers, and see if you can remember what you learn. It may also be helpful to take note or write any new information. Try to remember what the literature says is or are the reasons why an addict may relapse. Also, see if you can remember what the literature says is the chemical effect of the drugs in the literature review. Let us go to the literature. The general question psychologists ask is: "What is responsible for a relapse?"

Relapse is common in drug and alcohol recovery process. It is estimated that more than 90% of those with willingness to stay clean and sober have at least one relapse before they are able to stay clean and sober or achieve lasting recovery (Brady, 2012).

According to the literature, addiction may cause compulsive drug seeking and use, despite harmful consequences (NIDA, 2010). Being addicted means giving up conscious control. Addiction is a progressive disease that causes impulsive, unconscious behavior (Dean, 2009). When an individual is addicted to a substance such as alcohol, heroin, methamphetamine, marijuana, or prescription drugs, the individual is physically, mentally, or both physically and mentally dependent on the substance (Drug-Rehabs.org, 2009). In this chapter, the question we want to answer is what the literature says is the reason or reasons why individuals relapse or become dependent on street drugs and alcohol.

This is important to know from the literature in terms of existing studies before we go to the analysis and learn what the analysis will show is the reason or reasons or contributing factors to street drug and alcohol use and frequent relapse. Both the informations will be enriching and may lead to developing a new focus on drug and alcohol treatment.

Several approaches have been developed to decide or diagnose a person to be an addict. Some are basic and some complex. Some focus on question and answer with several variables to rule out by answering yes or no to questions designed for diagnosing addiction. Drawing from my years of experience working with individuals, groups, and cases on addiction, human behavior, prevention, and relapse, addiction may be defined as a physical, chemical, psychological dependence on drugs even when the individual is experiencing catastrophic problems from the drugs or behavior. There is another definition that considers addiction to be a brain disease. But, from experience I know, people with addiction problem may have different ways of describing what addiction is and what they look for in order to tell if a person is using or not using Drugs. This is why I came up with the following definition that addiction means being controlled, being attached to something, or an uncontrolled physical and chemical compulsion for drugs. If asked to diagnose a person, these are the signs or symptoms they look out for in making their judgment, and it may not be what the professional thinks or will use but is worth noting as follows: being skinny, always sneezing or coughing, have to have or got to have it, stealing, always broke, having red eyes, always looking around and hiding in fear of cops, body and feet odor due to poor hygiene, having an upset stomach, body rashes due to speed, anger and violence due to alcohol, and being homeless. Some of these signs may not have found their way into textbooks yet, but they may hold some meaningful insights into how addicts view their problems and symptoms. These may be the key to preventing another relapse. This is why it is important to check and not to let these pass by unnoticed. One caution is to avoid using the signs as stereotype and believing every person that exhibits one or two signs is using street drugs without taking into account a whole range of other related issues before a conclusion is drawn.

Addictive Drugs

Because the study involves the use of alcohol and drugs, three of the most common drugs and their effects are discussed in this section. Also, remember, drugs are not the only things people can be addicted to. There are different addictions. In this book, the author has only looked at chemical substances, including street drugs and alcohol addiction. The question you may ask is: Does all addiction have the same pattern? What pattern is common among all addictions? See if you can trace that from reading this book. Also, to learn the effect and multiple effects of each drug, you may need the information to compare with the information on drugs in chapter four. It is important to learn about the chemical impact of street drugs from individuals that used them just to have some comprehensive idea and also to see what part of the body is affected by different street drugs for prevention and minimizing risk to self or others. If certain drugs have the habit of increasing a person's anger level or rage or cause some psychotic problems or organ damage, clinicians may have useful information to take necessary steps to prevent the cause of foreseeable or unforeseeable problems to prevent relapse or refer for a clean health bill of rights just to know the status of the individual's system or his organ status. Why is this important? It is because trigger is not the only problem in drug and alcohol problem, let alone relapse behavior. There are chemical issues and the impact of long exposure of ingesting or using street drugs and alcohol on the individual's health and social system.

Methamphetamines

When an individual is under the influence of methamphetamines, and high doses are ingested, he or she may become aggressive or violent. Furthermore, there is intense but temporary anxiety resembling a panic disorder or generalized anxiety disorder, with paranoid and psychotic features. With higher doses, depressive episodes can occur and individuals may cause legal, family, or relational problems due to the influence of the drug (American Psychiatric Association [APA], 2004). They can experience altered mental and emotional behavior or exhibit maladaptive behavior.

Cocaine

In the case of cocaine dependence, users experience enhanced vigor shortly after use. They also experience: (a) gregariousness; (b) hyperactivity; (c) restlessness; (d) hypervigilance; (e) interpersonal sensitivity; (f) talkativeness; (g) anxiety; (h) tension; (i) alertness; (j) grandiose ideas; (k) anger; (l) impaired judgment; (m) elevated blood pressure; (n) perspiration and chills; (o) psychomotor problems; and (p) respiratory distress, such as chest pain, etc. (APA, 2004).

Alcohol

"Alcohol" is a generic name for a large group of organic chemical compounds (Boggan, 2008). According to Boggan, an alcoholic beverage is a drink that contains the chemical substance ethanol. Ethanol is the psychoactive constituent in an alcoholic beverage that affects the central nervous system. The effects of alcohol on humans and human behavior cannot be overemphasized. There are documented cases of alcohol's effects on cognition, behavior, and health. Alcohol is a central nervous system depressant that produces significant psychoactive effects (Reusch, n.d.).

Alcohol use has generated interest across the board because of its nature and the effect it has on users and nonusers (Boggan, 2008). A study conducted by the Harvard School of Public Health on college binge drinking in the 1990s documented evidence of the impact of alcohol on the behavior and mood of college students (Wechsler, Dowdall, Maenner, Gledhill-Hoyt, & Lee, 1998) (see Table 1).

It is estimated that 90% of the population of the United States has had some alcohol. Califano (2006) examined fifteen—to twenty-four-year-olds with alcohol-related problems. The study investigated alcohol-related violence, car crashes, and deaths among some students. Individuals with severe drug and alcohol problems failed to attain goals of typical development and psychosocial transition from adolescence to young adulthood, such as marriage, employment, financial independence, and educational attainment.

Table 1

Impact of Alcohol on the Mood and Behavior of College Students 1993-1997

Impact of alcohol	Percentage of students affected
Had study or sleep interrupted	60.6
Had to take care of a drunken student	50.2
Had been insulted or humiliated	28.6
Driving after drinking	35.8
Had experienced unwanted sexual advances	20.1
Argument with a friend	23.5
Damaged property	10.4
Missed a class	30.2

Addiction and Mental Illness

Drug and alcohol use affect mental health. Therefore, paying close attention to the drugs and mental health of the person is important. In the past, drug use and alcohol and mental health were kept separate. A patient would have to see a drug and alcohol counselor or therapist for behavior modification and dependence and see a psychiatrist for mental health problems like mood, psychosis, or thought disorder. But chemicals affect both mind and behavior. This is why present treatment seems to include both the problems under the term "co-occurring disorder or COD". Sometimes it is not as simple to judge as to which led to the other: Is it the drugs that led to mental health problems or is it the mental health problem that led to chemical dependence? This debate will continue, and you will have your own voice as to what you think it is. Also, rise in gun-related crimes against a person in the community whether they are drug, alcohol, mental illness, pure violence, anger, and social problems related requires new understanding of triggers in the community that may be potential for drug use, ongoing relapse, and any other behavior problem. Therefore, individuals with COD are "best served through an integrated screening, assessment, and treatment planning process that address both substance use and mental disorders, each in the context of the other" (CSAT, 2007, p. 1). Due to the complex nature of COD, screening, assessment, and treatment plans require flexibility rather than rigid plans. The CSAT (2007) has found:

> The complexity of COD dictates that screening, assessment, and treatment planning cannot be bound by a rigid formula. Rather, the success of this process depends on the skills and creativity of the clinician in applying available procedures, tools, and laboratory tests and on the relationships established with the client and his or her intimates. (p. 2)

The problem of COD and the treatment required is brought to view by the concerns around treatment challenges for this population. Sometimes, due to complexities of the nature of the problem, substance abuse and mental disorders, evidence of poor treatment outcomes within this group and the need for targeted treatment has been noted (CSAT, 2005). Also, according to CSAT, research has revealed that substance abusers with mental illness showed evidence of satisfactory outcomes with the use of traditional treatment methods for substance abuse. However, individuals with substance abuse issues concurrent with more serious mental disorders require modifications to the intervention program as well as supplementary programming to increase effectiveness of the program and result in successful outcomes (CSAT, 2005).

Chronic alcohol use, for example, has both a subtle and a dramatic impact on the brain and brain functioning. Ethanol affects sites in the human brain such as the cerebellum, involved in the coordination of bodily movements; the frontal cortex, primarily involved in the cognitive process; the occipital lobe, which contains the visual cortex; and part of the temporal lobe, involved in hearing (Boggan, 2008). In addition, increase in alcohol use increases psychiatric problems in young people suffering from depression, anxiety, defiance of authority, and antisocial personality disorders (Califano, 2006).

For this reason, problems of mental illness and substance abuse have gained the attention of California state drug and alcohol officials who want to see progress in COD treatment. In the fiscal year 1995-96 budget, the governor of California recognized that 60% of persons who had serious mental illness also had a substance abuse problem precipitating trouble with the law (California Department of Alcohol and Drug Programs, 2010). A closer look at the problem by the California Department of Alcohol and Drug Programs revealed that substance abuse treatment programs typically reported that 50-75% of their clients had COD, while corresponding mental health settings cited a proportion of 20-50% (California Department of Alcohol and Drug Programs Co-Occurring Disorders Unit, 2010).

Therefore, treating substance abuse requires not only putting intervention in place or immediately implementing group treatment but also an understanding of the experiences of individuals referred or sent into divergent program, going to treatment while jail is suspended, into treatment facilities from the community with pretreatment addiction relapse triggers should be studied for effective delivery of care and development of treatment goals and objectives. We have to think out of the box to develop the therapy model and analysis steps and also explain how this can be done at the same time an individual will be receiving psycho-educational group or individual therapy. Patton (2002) explained why the qualitative approach is a useful tool for analyzing addiction relapse trigger. Whether research data are more desirable, valid, or meaningful than self-reported data is not at issue; the fact is, therapists cannot observe what individuals have done in their pretreatment addiction phase and lifestyle before they are sent for treatment. Therefore, we must compile information on pretreatment addiction relapse triggers for understanding the nature, categories, patterns, and risks associated with pretreatment addiction relapse triggers after an individual relapses and before he or she is discharged back into the same community.

It makes a lot of sense why we should develop a treatment model and analysis steps to identify and analyze pretreatment addiction relapse triggers. The reason is: it is important to learn about addicts' thoughts and behavior before and after they became addicted. Recognizing the thought patterns and behaviors associated with addiction may help all stakeholders involved to go behind closed doors into the world of triggers contributing to drug and alcohol use (Chenail & Maione, 2009). Qualitative methodologies are powerful tools for enhancing our understanding of phenomenon such as unobserved addiction relapse triggers and behavior unseen by therapists (Hoepfl, 1997). While we all have opinions about why people use and what is the cause, we cannot know the full extent of the problem without research that will allow us to study pretreatment addiction relapse triggers to find out exactly what is driving every user to drug use and alcohol. Mind you, the problem of addiction triggers is not a problem of the poor; it is also a problem in most households and a problem of rich and poor and famous. Addiction has no boundaries. So we better develop the tool to identify and analyze it for effective treatment. With this in mind, we will move to a general understanding of the nature of triggers.

Triggers

As you read this section, see if you can learn what the literature says a trigger is and how is that different from your experience or personal definition. Also, find out if a trigger drives or influences behavior or feelings; if not, what does a trigger influence in an addict and why? It is very important you know what a trigger is and how it works, just to get the idea how it is affecting a real individual battling with the disease of addiction. The fact is clear that what triggers you may not trigger me, and sometimes we may carry the discussion further, asking if triggers are relative. A general understanding of triggers and how they affect individual users in research that has been completed will help pave the way when we move to the analysis section of this study. It is a step in the right direction and necessary for maximizing resources when helping individuals with relapse behavior problems. Why is this important? If you are not sure what the trigger is and what is driving the behavior or getting people to use drugs, alcohol, or prescription drugs over and over and relapse, you will be prompted to focus on changing or ending the behavior or thought. But that is not enough. Also, jail time may earn some addicts clean time, but that also will not be enough although it is better than now. We must go beyond the present traditional approach to treat individuals battling with the disease of addiction. What this means is that clinicians and policy makers first must be clear about finding the most effective and cost-less approach for understanding what is driving the relapse behavior and why. Every concerned counselor, therapist, and family member will want to know and find out what is causing the drug and alcohol use and relapse. Could it be availability of drugs, money, triggers, socioeconomic challenges, personality and psychological problems? If we accept the view that people are converting to drug and alcohol because of any or combination of the problems listed above, then we want to be scientific about it and test and rule out if liquor stores, availability, and access is the problem. Then, you are confronted with the next question of why are some going to get it when others are not? These sorts of questions may sound theoretical or open for debate, but finding an answer to them will maximize time, effort, resources, and save lives. You want to concentrate and pull in resources where you will have the maximum impact. The first thing you should understand about triggers is that triggers can cause stress, sadness, or glee ("Drug Addiction Triggers," 2010). In an effort to relieve sadness and stress, an addict may go in search of drugs. The drug, alcohol, or other substance makes addicts feel better at the time, and they come to associate those good feelings with the substance. Over time, the addicted person will begin to use the same substance whenever he or she wants to feel better ("Triggers," 2010). The most powerful triggers to avoid include particular people, places, and emotional triggers, such as thought, craving, and uses (USHHS, 2009).

Different kinds of triggers exist, including different environmental influences affecting addiction. These influences include family and friends, socio-community status, peer pressure, physical and sexual abuse, stress, parental involvement, and the critical developmental stages in a person's life that will cause or predispose a person to be vulnerable to drug use (NIDA, 2007).

The relationship between triggers and cues was demonstrated in Pavlov's classified conditioning paradigm within the realm of a dog's physiological response. In the experiment performed by Pavlov, the dogs became conditioned to salivate each time the bell rang and food was served (Carroll, 1998). After this conditioning was observed, the bell was rung, but no food was served (Carroll, 1998). The dogs continued to demonstrate the salivation response, even when the food was not served. It was concluded that this conditioned response resulted from the dogs being used to the sound of the bell and associating the food with the conditional cue of the bell (Carroll, 1998).

According to research, a similar effect has been observed in the human brain, which also learns to anticipate reaction to stimuli (Pate,

2009). As such, addiction relapse trigger has a similar effect in the part of the brain sensitive to external triggers. For example, people may experience overwhelming memories and emotions that seem to come out of nowhere when they hear music to which they used to get high, or pass by a street where they used to buy drugs or sex (Jaffe, 2010).

Triggers can cause relapse. A relapse trigger, like the bell in Pavlov's experiment, can be any person, place, thing, or situation that reminds a person of his or her drug and alcohol use (Urell, 2010). Common triggers include being around people with whom one previously used drugs, having money or getting paid, drinking alcohol, social situations, and certain affective states, such as anxiety, depression, or joy (Carroll, 1998).

Triggers and Addictive Behavior

Several studies have been done to investigate the relationship between triggers and addictive behavior in rats. Enkel, Spanagel, Vollmayr, and Schneider (2010) sought to determine whether stress or depression could trigger addiction in rats suffering from congenital helplessness or an accepted model of depression. The study also looked at whether increased or decreased consumption of a sweet solution under single-housing conditions could indicate anhedonia under stress. The researchers measured anhedonia by a reduction of sweetened condensed milk (SCM) intake.

According to Enkel et al. (2010), the rats in the study were kept in a single housing, which served as an environmental factor that induced anhedonia-like behavior in genetically predisposed rats. Thirty-two rats with depression, and thirty rats in the control group, aged nine to thirteen weeks, were used in the study. The rats were kept in a group-house in standard Macrolon cages and under standard conditions (twelve-hour light/dark cycle, lights on at 8:00 a.m.) with water and food available, except on testing day.

The animals were maintained on a mild food restriction timetable of 15 g lab chow per day. Furthermore, foot-shock stress exposure electric shocks were applied in modified Skinner boxes equipped with a grid floor consisting of twenty-four electrical steel rods and electrical walls. Levels were retracted. After three minutes of habituation, four unsignaled shocks (2 s, 0.8 mA, pulsed) were delivered at a variable interstimulus interval (60-30 s). One minute after the last shock, the rats were returned to the home cage. After five minutes of habituation, the rats had access to the sweetened solution for fifteen minutes. The amount of liquid consumed was recorded for each rat and was calculated in relation to the individual body weight (ml/kg).

The results of the study showed a reduction in milk intake among the helpless rats with anhedonia, compared to non-helpless rats, after the shock was administered. In addition, a decrease in PAS, indicating a deficient reward perception, was found. The results demonstrated that learned helplessness and stress trigger anhedonia-like behavior in congenitally helpless rats. Furthermore, stress shock can decrease milk consumption in rats with learned helplessness (Enkel et al., 2010). The study was limited in that other factors, like taste, could affect intake of milk.

Rajasekaram, Kumar, and Venkatachalam (2003) examined how the use of chemical substance increases the desire for continued use (i.e., whether the use of ingested chemicals increases the craving and use for more consumption). The substance used in the study by Rajasekaram et al. was neuronal nitric oxide syntheses (n NOS). The study investigated whether n NOS activity triggers picrotoxin-induced seizures or disorder of the nervous system as well as triggers increasing use of the substance at the same time. Adult male Wistar rats (150-170 g) were used throughout the study. The rats were housed in groups of three to four per cage and had free access to food and water under controlled temperatures (26-28°C) and light (12:12 day-night cycle). Controlled rats received PCT (5 mg/kg; 1. P). Thirty or sixty minutes were allowed before the administration of PCT. PCT-induced convulsive animals received 7-N1 (25 and 50 mg/kg, 1. P). NO-controlled rats received a saline solution.

The PCT-induced convulsive rats and the rats that received only the saline solution were evaluated. Animals were observed in individual Plexiglas boxes for sixty minutes after administration of PCT. The severity of seizure was graded as follows: facial and body tremors, myoclonic jerk of the whole body, clonic convulsion of the whole body, clonic-tonic convulsions with flexion of hind limbs, and clonic-tonic convulsions with extension of hind limbs. Animals were exterminated prior to the onset of stage three seizure (i.e., eleven minutes after injection of PCT). The brains were quickly dissected into five regions:

frontal cortex, hippocampus, cerebellum, medullas, and the rest of the brain, including the thalamus and hypothalamus.

The data were analyzed using the student *t*-test and ANOVA, followed by Turkey's multiple companion tests, with P values less than 0.05, which were considered statistically significant. The results showed that rats with a PCT dose of 5 mg/kg exhibited all seizure stages, while rats with the 7-NI response delayed the onset of stage three seizures. DIA was determined to be the threshold of anticonvulsant doses required to prevent the expression of stage five seizures.

Sociological and Environmental Triggers

Sociological and environmental triggers influence the way we think, feel, behave, respond, and react in any given situation. What may trigger an individual to respond in this way or that way depends on many variables, but sociological and environmental triggers may play a part in cases of individual behavior.

Specific environmental and social factors may serve as triggers for individuals who have completed substance abuse treatment and returned to their previous environment and social circumstances. Rosenbloom (2009) conducted a study on triggers designed to test holiday willpower and drug and alcohol dependence. Holidays are particularly perilous times for those in treatment for alcohol problems; naltrexone has been suggested as an aid to help avoid alcohol-related problems. Medications work only if the patients take them, and the holidays are the worst time for patients' willpower, so these often dramatically fail (Rosenbloom, 2009).

The data showed that patients were reluctant to use available resources to mitigate holiday stress and triggers well before the holiday, resulting in relapse. Rosenbloom (2009) suggested that therapists should proactively recommend naltrexone as an aid to treatment, providing an extra insurance, rather than lament the challenges after the fact.

Early maturation, family problems, and poverty are also possible triggers for drug and alcohol use (Costello, Sung, Worthman, & Angold, 2006; Rosenbloom, 2009). Adolescent substance use and abuse have been linked to a wide range of family and environmental problems (Costello et al., 2006). Costello et al. tested the theory that puberty exacerbates triggers for drug use. The authors aggregated a large number of risk factors included in the test data set into three categories, using item response modeling and factor analysis. The group labeled "poverty and adversity" included: (a) family income below the federal poverty line; (b) parental lack of education; (c) parental unemployment; (d) single, step, and adopted family structure; and (e) multiple moves of home and school. The group labeled "family problems" showed: (a) parental history of mental illness; (b) crime; (c) drug problems; and (d) family violence and other risk factors, including childhood psychiatric disorders, life events, and association with deviant peers.

Statistical analysis showed that increased age predicted increased likelihood of alcohol use (Costello et al., 2006). Costello et al. reported that increased levels of testosterone were associated with risks of alcohol use in boys, controlling for age. From age 12 onward, mature boys had higher rates of alcohol risk than did immature boys. Among girls, the interaction was not significant. Mature girls had a higher alcohol risk than immature girls after age 12. The link between early maturation and conduct disorder was seen in girls only. Of maturing girls, 80% had conduct disorder and deviant peers using alcohol. For maturing boys, the percentage was 83%. The increased risk of alcohol use associated with all three risk factors was significant for both boys and girls.

The results of the study by Costello et al. (2006) demonstrated that family triggers such as early maturity, family poverty, and adversity did not increase the risk of alcohol use in early-maturing boys or girls. Interestingly, poverty marginally decreased the risk of alcohol use among early maturing boys; however, child-rearing style, specifically the lack of adequate supervision, increased the risk of alcohol use for both. Family problems increased the risk of alcohol use in early-maturing boys, but the effect on girls, while in the same direction, was not significant. The impact of early maltreatment (neglect, physical abuse, or sexual abuse) on boys was not a significant trigger, and although girls who had been maltreated reached maturity on average eight months earlier than non-maltreated girls, early maltreatment had no effect on alcohol use in girls. When the interrelation of different family risk factors was tested to predict early alcohol use for early-maturing girls, the results showed that the risk was present and increased for girls. Finally, Costello et al. concluded that although poverty was a marker for boys in terms of risk for use of alcohol, poverty was not a significant risk factor for girls' use of alcohol.

Many of us may come from homes that are not master of good parental knowledge, skills, and stability. The insecurity and instability created in these kinds of homes could drive a same person on the edge to look for support and coping outside the parental environment. This is because many homes are not suited to teach relationship. Some children due to in-home environmental instability and daily environmental stress will run away if it is an adult spends a lot of time away from home and shows up only to sleep. In this kind of environment, it does not matter it could be a religious or political environment that is very toxic, how do folks cope with environmental parental care and family stress or leadership stress? A study that looked at this problem investigates the relationship between parental support and alcohol use. Experience has revealed that some individuals claimed they started their drug and alcohol use very early in life as children growing up at home where they are exposed to chemical substance, alcohol or drugs, from age 7. Most have had their first experience before age 18. Parents' drinking behavior and favorable attitudes about alcohol, as well as lack of parental support, monitoring, and communications, have contributed to frequent drinking behavior, including heavy drinking and drunkenness in adolescence. Also, peer drinking and peer acceptance affect a significant number of adolescents and young adults between ages 12 and 20, though drinking under age 21 is illegal (Califano, 2006). Califano also found that adolescents who start drinking before age 15 are four times more likely to develop alcohol dependence than those who begin drinking at age 21; therefore, by the time an adolescent turns seventeen or eighteen years of age and is ready for college, he or she may have already developed a drinking problem.

Tevyaw, Borsari, Colby, and Monti (2007) designed a study to determine the effectiveness of incorporating peer motivation for decreasing alcohol use among college students mandated to receive treatment after violating campus alcohol policy. In the study, thirty-six male participants were randomly assigned to receive either two 45-minute sessions of an individual motivational intervention (IMI, $n = 18$) or a peer-enhanced motivational intervention (PMI, $n = 18$). The IMI variables included: (a) exploration of motivation to change alcohol use; (b) perceived negative effect of drinking; (c) personalized feedback; and (d) goals for changing alcohol consumption and related behaviors. The PMI variables included all elements or variables of the

IMI plus the presence of a supportive peer of the participants during both sessions.

The results provided by Tevyaw et al. (2007) showed that the magnitude of within-group reduction in alcohol use and problems was three times larger on average for the PMI than for the IMI group. Therefore, the findings reported by Tevyaw et al. showed promise for the inclusion of peers in brief motivational intervention for mandated students as a future strategy for reducing alcohol behaviors.

The limitation of the study by Tevyaw et al. (2007) is that it failed to account for environmental problems and predisposing factors that may contribute to drinking behavior and drunkenness among college students. The usefulness of the study is that peer influence could help decrease alcohol use if included in treatment intervention. Keep in mind the study cited among college students in a college or learning environment in Table 1, *Impact of Alcohol on the Mood and Behavior of College Students 1993-1997. It showed,* among other things, behaviors such as oversleeping, insult, drunk driving, unwanted sexual advances, argument, damage to property, and missed classes. The question is: What is responsible for violence against a person or property? Could alcohol, drugs, and social environment or triggers in the environment be responsible for violence against a person or damage to property? What cautionary steps should be taken to monitor an individual's social environment triggers and drug access to prevent unforeseen violent behavior against any person and property damage? These questions are questions of fact not opinions. Also, they are questions of relationship or to determine whether triggers in the environment may cause relapse behavior? Up until now, the need to focus drug and alcohol treatment on pretreatment addiction relapse triggers has not been a major focus in addiction treatment, because the psychotherapy model and analysis steps for doing this kind of work has not been developed. Also, a lot of therapy emphasis with some exceptions has been cognitive behavior modification than tracking and analysis of triggers. But this focus is interesting and important if we want to make a big difference in addiction triggers. Therefore, a theoretical framework, a therapy model for identifying, and steps for analyzing pretreatment addiction relapse trigger risk has to be developed. The reason being, it is not just enough to say a person has experienced triggers, but it has to be shown and presented scientifically, including on ongoing risk.

This is the focus of this book, and the author has made a contribution to the study of addiction triggers by developing qualitative therapy and analysis steps for trigger identification, analysis, and risk identification. We will not shift our attention to laying the theoretical foundation used in developing a qualitative or a Q therapy model and analysis presented in this book for understanding pretreatment addiction relapse trigger. First, we will look at qualitative research theory as the starting point for understanding qualitative therapy, patient care in and out of treatment. The author's core mission for writing about qualitative therapy and analysis steps is to bring the next generation of addiction therapy model, knowledge, skills, and scientific technique readily accessible for identifying pretreatment addiction relapse trigger, analysis, and risk level and benefit from a cutting-edge scientific approach. The aim is to bring focus on pretreatment addiction relapse trigger and science to trigger identification, analysis, and risk level analysis to improve qualitative therapy model and analysis works and is a very effective method for pretreatment addiction relapse trigger identification and analysis that has the potential of becoming a broad new clear addiction treatment approach to demonstrate scientifically possible risk of pretreatment addiction relapse trigger to patients. We are not charging for the knowledge because the author's interest is to make information available to improve life. The information on qualitative therapy model and analysis steps has the ability to utilize the best of science in addiction treatment at no cost.

Qualitative Research Methods for Clinicians

The benefit of qualitative research cannot be overemphasized. The author, as a clinician, has developed qualitative therapy or Q therapy for use in Education for Recovery in Addiction group by adopting steps in qualitative research in group process. The justification for developing a therapy patterned after qualitative research approach and analysis steps is qualitative research and produces findings not obtained by statistical procedures or other means of quantification (Neill, 2009). Qualitative research approach has been used to study phenomenon of any kind. Because of this possibility, qualitative research methods offer a great possibility if adapted to addiction treatment to improve potential for understanding pretreatment addiction relapse trigger, a topic rarely understood for it categories, patterns, and risk levels and implication in addiction treatment. Therapists have a choice to keep using and staying on what general information on triggers is available, using the present treatment therapy model, but for more in-depth identification and analysis of trigger categories, patterns, and risk levels, the qualitative research method offers great potential for understanding pretreatment addiction relapse triggers beyond theoretical nuance. Therefore, instead of constructing theories, as their researcher colleagues have done, researching clinicians must: (a) face their previous constructions (sense-making from experience); (b) create methods that allow for deconstruction (sense-making challenged); and then (c) work toward building reconstructions (sense-making remade) (Chenail & Maione, 2009).

Also, the use of qualitative research methods for data analysis can have several benefits. Clinicians can reflect on one observation at a time and use a new sense-making perspective to look for something qualitatively different in the phenomenon from what is known and from what had been the focus of study (Chenail & Maione, 2009). Qualitative research creates the atmosphere for developing an understanding of situations or problems like the one covered in this study and analysis, pretreatment addiction relapse triggers prior to the change factor or prior to the time skills are applied.

Qualitative Analysis of Addiction

Qualitative methods have been used in drug and alcohol research for developing an understanding of triggers and relapse and for studying the impact of drug and alcohol use in a sociocultural context (Sterk-Elifson, 1995), except in Education for Recovery in Addiction group process and analysis presented in this report. Sterk-Elifson examined changes in drug-use patterns and the impact of drug-use patterns on women's lives and on related issues such as support of the drug habit and setting of use. The project was called "Project Fast," and the duration of the study was between June 1992 and June 1994.

The study utilized in-depth interviewing of the women, supplemented by ethnographic or social mapping, including participant observation, with the researchers visiting the women in different neighborhoods and interviewing them (Sterk-Elifson, 1995). The criteria used to determine eligibility was that female participants must live in the Atlanta metropolitan area, be eighteen years of age or older, and be active drug users, where the term "active drug user" was defined as injecting on at least four days per week during the last year (Sterk-Elifson, 1995). Crack cocaine users had to use at least three grams of cocaine per week or use daily during the last year (Sterk-Elifson, 1995).

A total of 164 female drug users participated in the study. The women were interviewed about topics such as family background; reproduction history; drug use and drug treatment experience; violence; abuse; and health history, including HIV and AIDS. In addition to the interview data, a focus group provided another level of analysis and consensus building. Rather than forming a process group, Sterk-Elifson (1995) conducted in-depth interviews, supplemented by ethnographic contact with the addicts. Qualitative measures included demographic characteristics, such as self-esteem and knowledge of HIV and AIDS.

Women in the focus groups discussed and provided insight into their triggers and experiences. The data revealed the triggers, behaviors, and patterns of drug use among the women in the Atlanta area who participated in the study. The data were critical for understanding substance abuse patterns and for developing intervention strategies to minimize potential harm from drug use to the users, users' communities, and society at large (Sterk-Elifson, 1995).

Qualitative Analysis of Recovery, Relapse, and Prevention

Relapse after drug and alcohol treatment may be related to genetic factors, changes in neurons and neurotransmitter function from heavy use, and the continuance of these changes within the brain after cessation of use, enabling environmental triggers to cause craving and relapse. It is necessary for any method designed to prevent or minimize relapses to consider the individual triggers and stressors (Kelly et al., 2007). Kelly et al. reported:

Relapses are not sudden events that fall out of the blue. Patients need to learn the chains of events and behaviors that lead to their relapses. Triggers and stresses are often highly individual. They must be identified in each person in order to help him or her learn to prevent or minimize relapses. (p. 381)

Harris, Fallot, and Berley (2005) used qualitative semi-structured interviews to examine elements of sustained recovery among women with COD who had survived trauma, with a focus on substance abuse recovery. They asked twenty-seven women to describe the most significant factors in both sustaining and hindering their recovery. Harris et al. identified seven themes in the factors that sustained or hindered the recovery of participants; four of these were supportive, and three served as obstacles to recovery. Connection, self-awareness, a sense of purpose and meaning, and spirituality were listed as supportive themes revealed through the analysis, whereas battles with depression and despair, destructive habits and patterns, and lack of personal control were revealed as themes that were obstacles to recovery.

Smith (2006) explored chronic sorrow as a relapse trigger for female substance abusers with a history of child abuse who were enrolled in a substance abuse treatment program for relapse. Smith utilized qualitative measures to describe the participants' feelings and experiences related to their relapse. According to Smith, twelve women participated in semi-structured interviews to explore their perceptions of relapse. The findings of the study revealed three common themes: (a) mothering loss; (b) blocking feelings; and (c) relapse triggers. Participants suggested the use of interpersonal reflection as well as cognitive and action-based coping skills as a means of avoiding relapse.

Psychosocial interventions characteristically maintain a focus on both abstinence and personal and social coping mechanisms (Kelly et al., 2007). Cognitive-behavioral therapy (Beck, 1993) underscores the need to understand a person's false beliefs (cognitive element) that may have precipitated the substance use and abuse; with this understanding, the patient is able to change the way he or she deals with the craving and avoid using the addictive substance (behavioral element). The therapist works with the patient to employ behavioral changes to avoid the addictive behavioral response (Kelly et al., 2007).

Motivational interviewing (Miller & Rollnick, 2009) is a method in which the therapist leads the addict through several stages of change.

Miller and Rollnick state: "Motivational interviewing is a collaborative, person-centered form of guiding to elicit and strengthen motivation for change" (p. 137). The stages range from unawareness of the need for change from substance dependence, to a realization of the need to change, to taking action to change behaviors, to finally maintaining behavioral changes. The therapist focuses on the individual's personal motivations for change and incorporates them into the behavioral change implementation plan. Within this strategy, relapse is accepted as possible, yet not a failure. Instead, a relapse signals the need to move backward in the stages, without erosion of the individual's self-efficacy (Kelly et al., 2007).

The development of an acceptance-based coping intervention designed to prevent alcohol dependency relapse was presented by Vieten et al. (2010), who contended that negative effect serves as a common relapse trigger after successful treatment for alcohol dependency. Vieten et al. presented an intervention strategy unique from the change-based strategies commonly used for managing negative affect (or cognitions), termed *Acceptance-Based Coping for Relapse Prevention (ABCRP)*. ABCRP was designed to treat alcohol-dependent individuals within the first six months of initial and continued abstinence from drinking.

Qualitative Analysis of Addiction Among Forensic Mentally Ill

Bradizza and Stasiewicz (2003) designed a study to analyze high-risk drug and alcohol use situations among severely mentally ill-substance abusers. According to Bradizza and Stasiewicz, situational factors have been found to influence relapse to alcohol and drug use in general samples of abuse; however, little research exists that examines the influence of interpersonal and intrapersonal determinants in samples of individuals dually diagnosed with severe mental illness (SMI) and substance use disorders (SUI). The Bradizza and Stasiewicz study was designed to obtain qualitative data from the participants regarding the types of high-risk alcohol and drug-use situations they most often encountered in their daily lives. The study represented the first known effort to assess higher risk situations in SMI.

The study by Bradizza and Stasiewicz (2003) assessed high-risk alcohol and drug-use situations in dually diagnosed individuals, using focus group data. Bradizza and Stasiewicz developed a taxonomy of relapse episodes, based on interviews with abusers who emphasized a situational analysis of potential relapse episodes. Relapse episodes were classified into one of eight types of intrapersonal and interpersonal situations. The interpersonal situations included unpleasant emotional states, pleasant emotions, physical discomfort, testing personal control, and urges or temptations to use. The interpersonal situations included conflict with others, social pressure to use, and pleasant times with others.

In the Bradizza and Stasiewicz (2003) study, the individuals who participated (twenty-one women and twenty men) were diagnosed primarily with a psychotic disorder or a recurrent major affective disorder. The study was conducted using the following methods: Participants were recruited from two dual-diagnosis outpatient programs in the Buffalo, New York area. The participants were 75% African American, 19% Caucasian, and 6% Hispanic; 72% were single or never married, 25% were separated or divorced, and 3% were married or cohabiting. Participants had a mean 11.3 years of education, and 94% were currently unemployed. Fifty-five percent had a major affective disorder diagnosis (44% major depression, 8% bipolar, 3% dysthymia), and 45% had a psychotic disorder diagnosis (22% schizophrenia, 17% schizoaffective, 6% psychotic disorder NOS). Psychotic medication was being prescribed for 97% of participants.

According to Bradizza and Stasiewicz (2003), data for analysis were collected from a focus group discussion and from patient charts. The medical charts were reviewed at the clinic, and information was obtained regarding demographic mental health, substance abuse diagnosis, and psychiatric medication. The group data were typed, rather than handwritten or typed, and later transcribed for analysis.

Bradizza and Stasiewicz (2003) described the data collection process for the study as follows: The group was asked questions about difficulties in handling everyday situations; questions focused on alcohol and drug use. The group session began with questions regarding general social situations they found difficult to manage. They were also asked about high-risk situations or triggers for substance abuse. Participants were required to attend one of ten 75-minute audiotaped sessions. The groups were small, with only six to twelve individuals, and the sessions were facilitated by a group moderator, who gave the members final opportunities to contribute.

The data obtained for the study, according to Bradizza and Stasiewicz (2003), were divided into two parts: numbers and descriptive statistics were used to analyze the qualitative demographic and diagnosis information obtained from the chart review, and qualitative data was analyzed through the use of a multilevel process that focused on the classification of responses related to high risk during an alcohol use situation. The results showed a consensus of ten themes encompassing a total of thirty-three higher risk situations. These themes included both interpersonal and intrapersonal situations. Each of the themes was extracted from the data. The study demonstrated that qualitative research techniques offer insight into understanding the behavior of participants and provide a valuable foundation for further quantitative study. The study also showed that individuals with SMI can participate in semi-structured focus groups. Understanding the mentality and behavior associated with addiction could help everybody involved in treatment gain knowledge that exists behind closed doors and find unobserved pretreatment relapse triggers within a world of secrets and addiction (Chenail & Maione, 2009).

Models for Treating Addiction

This is important. We cannot talk about street drugs, triggers and addiction without talking about treatment. How do we understand addiction influence treatment planning? As a family member, with a loved one under the influence, finding the right kind of treatment is important, but what is most important is first finding an understanding about addiction and the models of treatment. There are existing conceptual models for understanding and treating addicts and addiction. Psychotherapy models are supported by theoretical understanding of a problem in this case, addiction. Also, models are ways people think about what a problem is about and what to do or how to treat or respond to the problem. For example, in the moral model, alcohol problems are viewed as willful violations of social rules and norms. Therefore, moral and social sanctions are important interventions. The addict is seen as the problem, making bad choices.

Temperance Model

In the temperance model, alcohol is believed to be a very dangerous drug that people should avoid at all costs. Those using spiritual models perceive alcohol dependency as a condition people are powerless to overcome without turning their lives and asking for help from a higher power.

Disease Model

Within the disease models, addiction is viewed as a disease, irreversible, and incapable of being cured. Therefore, a person with the condition should be identified, diagnosed, and treated.

Educational Model

In the educational model, alcohol problems are viewed as evolving from deficient knowledge or lack of accurate information. Therefore, this model combines education or providing information to individuals by teaching and skill training to influence negative belief with positive belief to influence behavior. Therefore, the application of cognitive behavior therapy has played a dominant role within the educational model.

Cognitive models emphasize the need to convert mental processes, converting positive expectation about use of drugs and alcohol into guiding behavior. Biological models understand addiction as an inherited brain physiological problem that requires genetic counseling and medical treatment.

Character Logical Model

The character model addiction is a dysfunction within a person's personality traits and defense mechanisms. Therefore, psychotherapy is the best intervention. Psychosocial and behavior treatment can include skill training and a variety of counseling approaches including individual or group counseling (House of Rep. February, 2000).

The Psychological Model

Psychological model drug and alcohol is a problem that originates from a dysfunction of three sources: motivational, learning, or emotional dysfunction. Also, addiction problems may be symptoms of psychopathology (intra-psychic conflict) or social learning problems (behavioral model).

Behavioral Model

The behavioral model states people use drugs only to relieve distress associated with depression, hyperactivity, restlessness, and bipolar illness.

Social Learning-Based Model

The social learning-based models state that people use drugs because of social deficits and cognitive coping skills that lead to an inability to manage everyday stress. Social learning model treatment tools include individual and psychotherapy or group therapy.

Sociocultural Model

The sociocultural model states that addiction is a direct result of lifelong socialization processes within addiction-promoting social and cultural environments. Treatment tools include environmental restructuring that provides living arrangements and involvement with self-help groups.

Residential Treatment Model

The residential treatment model is the vehicle for intensive treatment of inmates with drug and alcohol problems. It includes both inpatient (500 hours of treatment over six to twelve months) and outpatient treatment, multiple weekly contacts with peer support groups, family or couple therapy, treatment contracts, abstinence activities, urine monitoring, and education and individual psychotherapy. Inpatient treatment consists of two phases of treatment. In phase one, the therapist assesses inmates' skills of interpersonal communication, cognitive processing, and decision making, as well as the history of drug and alcohol use, consequences, and medical problems, and education on psychopharmacology and varying theories on addiction. In phase two, inmates confront deficits identified during the initial phase, allowing inmates to focus on personal strengths and weaknesses.

According to a report published by the National Center on Addiction and Substance Abuse of Columbia University in March 2003, 80% of all offenders in the US Criminal Justice system report having substance abuse problems (Bureau of Justice Assistance, 2005). Thus, the need for drug treatment in state federal prison and local jails is evident.

Resident Substance Abuse Treatment for State Prisoners Program, or RSAT, was created to help states and local governments develop, implement, and improve residential substance abuse treatment programs in state and local correctional and detention facilities (Bureau of Justice Assistance, April 2005). It creates and maintains community-based aftercare services for probationers and parolees, in addition to programs within secure settings that help offenders overcome their substance abuse problems and prepare for reentry into society. The program provides staff and resources to address all aspects of substance abuse behavior, allowing inmates to focus on their recovery (Bureau of Justice Assistance, 2005). Congress established the RSAT program under the Violent Crime Control and Law Enforcement Act of 1994 (pub. 103-322, 1901).

A state may use RSAT grant funds to implement one of four types of programs: state and local correctional facility RSAT programs, jail-based treatment programs, aftercare programs, and post-release treatment programs (Bureau of Justice Assistance, 2005). Participants should have between six and twelve months left to serve out their sentences at the time of entry into the program, so they can be released from prison after they complete the program. The program should provide resident treatment such as living in apartments separate from the general correctional population in either a separated facility or a dedicated housing unit used exclusively for the program (Bureau of Justice Assistance, 2005).

The RSAT treatment programs are designed to focus on inmates' cognitive behavior, social behavior, and skills to solve the substance abuse and other related problems. The program includes the use of urine analysis or other reliable forms of drug and alcohol testing. It is further recommended that individuals released from the RSAT program, who remain in the custody of a state or local government, should also continue to be tested (Bureau of Justice Assistance, 2005).

RSAT programs in prisons and jails educate inmates about substance abuse, including the consequence of the addiction cycle, recovery, the relationship of alcohol and drug abuse to their problems, and how to work through denial and blaming of others for their drug abuse problems. Programs help participants understand behaviors such as anger, criminal behavior, poor skills, and habit development. Offenders are taught how to control anger, manage their stress and emotions, resolve conflicts, and set goals and boundaries.

In addition, RSAT program may help participants develop social, communication, and coping skills. Some programs reinforce positive behavior rather than focusing on negative behavior. RSAT programs may also include twelve-step programs such as Alcoholic Anonymous or Narcotics Anonymous (Bureau of Justice Assistance, 2005). A popular treatment model is *Thinking for a Change*, an integrated cognitive behavior curriculum that concentrates on cognitive restructuring and developing social and problem-solving skills (Bureau of Justice Assistance, 2005).

Also, some RAST are designed to be gender responsive treatment to women. Programs that are designed for women address women issues and educate women and girls about self-esteem, self-sufficiency, and wellness, discussing topics such as codependent relationships and eating disorders. Many programs include components that address parenting and family issues, such as domestic violence, relationships, and communication. Family therapy may be offered (Bureau of Justice Assistance, 2005).

California's total funding for RSAT programs was over 44 million dollars ($44, 086,489). This money was used in funding programs for adult male and female juvenile inmates in California. In all, 9,762 offenders successfully completed an RSAT-funded program. During 2002, California had five RSAT projects representing four sites, at which a total of 3,752 offenders completed treatment (Bureau of Justice Assistance, 2005).

Cognitive Behavioral Therapy Treatment

Before we make any further move to describe why the author thinks qualitative therapy will offer more scientific advantage in drug and alcohol treatment because it was discovered and developed out of a crushing need in the Inland Empire of California to address the issue and topic of pretreatment addiction relapse trigger by psychoeducational group process and scientific analysis of pretreatment addiction relapse trigger that otherwise would have been impossible without the discovery and development by the author. But first, it will be informative to discuss the present therapy model widely in use in drug treatment, cognitive behavior therapy or CBT.

Cognitive Behavior Therapy (CBT) was developed by Aaron T. Beck at the University of Pennsylvania in the 1960s (Beck, 1995). The goal is directed toward solving current problems and modifying dysfunctional thinking and behavior (Beck, 1995). The literature on drug and alcohol treatment seems to mention cognitive-behavioral therapy as the overwhelming psychological theoretical approach used in drug and alcohol treatment. The US Department of Health and Human Services Manual One stated that more than twenty years of research has shown that addiction is clearly treatable (Carroll, 1998). The manual utilized CBT as a short-term, focused approach to helping cocaine-dependent individuals become abstinent from cocaine and other substances (Carroll, 1998). The manual explained why CBT should be used in treatment because CBT is designed to help patients learn to recognize, avoid, and cope with issues and problems in their personal lives. Cognitive behavior therapy is structured, goal oriented, and focused on the immediate problems faced by cocaine abusers entering treatment who are struggling to control their cocaine use; yet CBT is a flexible, individualized approach that can be adapted to a wide range of patients as well as a variety of settings (impatient, outpatient) and formats (group, individual). The CBT approach has been extensively evaluated in rigorous clinical trials and has solid empirical support as treatment for cocaine abuse (Carroll, 1998).

Cognitive behavioral therapy has two components. First, functional analysis is used to help patients early in the treatment process assess and determine high-risk situations that are likely to lead to cocaine use and to provide insight into some of the reasons the individual may be using cocaine. Also, functional analysis helps individuals identify those situations or states in which the individual continues to have difficulty coping later in treatment (Carroll, 1998). The second component is the skill training aspect. Here, individuals receive training on how to unlearn old habits associated with cocaine abuse and learn or relearn healthier skills and habits.

It is assumed that individual skills to prevent relapse may be most effective initially but become less effective due to relapse over a period of time. Therefore, the individual needs to continue to learn new skills. Cognitive behavioral therapy also addresses several tasks, including motivation for abstinence, teaching coping skills, and changing reinforcement by identifying and reducing habits associated with drug-use lifestyle by substituting more enduring positive activities and rewards (Carroll, 1998). Individuals are taught skills to respond to painful events such as urges, depression, and anger. Also, individuals are taught to expand their social support and build enduring, drug-free relationships. Cognitive-behavioral therapy is a general therapeutic approach used in treatment of addiction to modify negative or self-defeating thoughts and behaviors, changing both thought and behavior (Sacks & Ries, 2005).

Cognitive behavior therapy is an alternative treatment or supplemental approach that allows observation and descriptive analyses of rich phenomena of individual experiences of addiction and relapse to make treatment decisions. When used in group settings, CBT creates possibilities for sharing and exploring ideas, including patterns of assumption such as thought, belief, cognition, insight, and judgment, that influenced thought, feelings, cravings, and behaviors of individuals in treatment. Cognitive behavior therapy also explores schemas developed in early life that form part of ones cultural and biological development. Cognitive behavior therapy is used for observation, testing, analyzing, and explaining a phenomenon in order to understand the phenomena as completely as the one telling the story.

The goal of cognitive treatment approach is to understand individual thoughts and feelings and how each impacts behavior with the hope of changing behavior through influence of changing the mind.

This process of changing subconscious thoughts is called cognitive restructuring. There is a general assumption that people initiate certain behaviors based on their belief and thought patterns. Cognitive therapy is used in group settings to learn how to refute distortions of fact. Cognitive restructuring theory states that unrealistic beliefs generate dysfunctional emotions and behaviors. Cognitive behavior therapy has been used in a number of different ways to treat individuals with depression, anxiety, and post-traumatic stress disorder and was later used in treating individuals with alcohol—and drug-related problems.

A second application of CBT aims at treating fear that develops in response to panic attacks with agrophobia. Agrophobia consists of multiple and varied fears and avoidance behavior that centers on the fear of leaving home and the fear of being alone.

A third application CBT aims at reducing symptoms associated with generalized panic attacks. Typically during a panic attack, a patient will be engaged in a routine activity like reading a book, eating in a restaurant, driving a car, or attending a concert when he or she will experience a sudden onset of overwhelming fear, terror, apprehension, and a sense of impending doom.

Several other symptoms are associated with panic attacks, such as physical palpitation, chest pain, choking or smothering sensations, dizziness or unsteadiness, feelings of unreality (serialization), hot and cold flushes, sweating, trembling, shaking, as well as fear of dying, going crazy, or losing control of oneself. It is clear that the above physical sensations of panic attacks represent massive overstimulation of the autonomic nervous system. Symptoms will last for five to twenty minutes but rarely as long as an hour.

Cognitive behavior therapy application aims at reducing symptoms by breath training, to control both acute and chronic hyperventilation, and exposure to somatic cures. Somatic cures usually involve a hierarchy of exposure to feared sensations through imaginary and behavioral exercises and relaxation. As such, CBT involves cognitive restructuring aimed at providing a more benign intervention for the uncomfortable effects and physical sensations associated with panic attacks or agrophobia. The assumption is that although panic attacks or fear trigger extreme physical sensations such as burst of tachycardia, they can still help themselves to a significant degree by changing the interpretation of these events from one thought process to another.

A fourth application of CBT falls in treating veterans with post-traumatic stress disorder (PTSD). The primary approach to treating PTSD includes exposure to avoid thoughts, feelings, images, and other stimuli with the aim of reducing associated symptoms. In PTSD treatment studies, the exposure method is typically used either alone or with other cognitive behavioral procedures to reduce avoidance, fear, and anxiety, and to challenge PTSD-related irrational thoughts (Lombardo, 2005). Lombardo contended that combat veterans could have other problems that exposure can help. Therefore, treatment alternatives for soldiers with PTSD should have multi-components that include flexible administered social and emotional skills training with exposure to improve outcome of combat veterans. In reference to treating veterans with PTSD and alcohol or drug-related problems, Lombardo (2005) suggested that researchers and clinicians should routinely screen substance abuses, apply imaginable and in vitro exposure plus coping skills training (Lombardo, 2005).

Several treatment models have been developed over time to treat clients with drug and alcohol problems. While existing therapy models may have their usefulness in terms of contributing to addiction treatment, we still need a specific therapy model with the ability to use or adapt research processes and scientific analysis to identify and analyze pretreatment addiction relapse triggers, which for most part goes under the radar. Any such therapy should improve clinical capability through scientific analysis and presentation categories, patterns, and risk of pretreatment addiction relapse trigger, a major barrier in patient achieving sobriety and staying clean and sober without relapsing. The consequence of recidivism, repeated relapse or exposure to chemicals from street drugs and alcohol ingestion, cannot be overstated on the victim's overall system, organ function, mental, social and spiritual health, preventing them from making meaningful contribution to the society. The issue of drug and alcohol addiction and chemical exposure cannot be overemphasized, pass by unnoticed, or be a legal matter only. It is society issue and for most part life and death issue for the user prolong use and exposure to poisonous chemicals and damage to organ function and also to victim killed by a person under the influence wielding a gun. Some of you may be familiar with or have direct first-hand information to share. This is why the appeal of Dine et al. for effective and urgent treatment approach cannot be passed by unnoticed and is needed and necessary (Dine et al., 1993). According to Dine, the recommended drug and alcohol treatment should focus on biological, psychological, and sociocultural issues. The biological approach is a medical model that describes alcohol's prolonged use or dependence as a progressive disease requiring treatment and supervision by medical staff. The psychological model looks at addiction problems from psychopathology (intra-psychic conflict) or social learning (behavioral model).

The present recommended treatment drug and alcohol treatment should incorporate a variety of rehabilitative services (e.g., housing, education vocational training, medical services, and child care). Also, drug and alcohol treatment approaches should seek to target the biological, psychological, and sociocultural dimensions of clients (Nunes et al., 1993). The biological treatment approach is a medical model that describes addiction as a progressive disease requiring medication treatment and supervision by medical staff.

The biological treatment has two main outcomes: first, the client is to withdraw from the addictive stimulus by the conventional detoxification approach and by environmental measures which include: alternate residence, altering client's access to money, curtailing social activities, changing client's phone number, providing alternate activities to drug use and monitoring of visits. The second goal is to prevent relapse. Well-accepted techniques for enhancing resilience to relapse include predicting situations in which relapse risk is higher, rehearsing avoidance strategies, changing lifestyle, developing a drug-free network, and reflecting negative consequences of abuse.

Although use of most drugs may show decrease during and after treatment, we should not forget that relapse is also common immediately after treatment or when a patient is released or discharged into the community he or she relapsed from and was arrested from before being sent to jail and a divergent treatment program that suspended them from serving time in jail without treatment. There is the possibility that relapse could be delayed if a combination of treatment models and approaches are initiated during both inpatient and outpatient treatment. Also, the use of reasonable action therapy with CBT could delay relapse in patients with PTSD, anxiety disorders, and alcohol and drug problems.

How Effective Is CBT?

CBT can be thought of as a highly individualized training program that helps cocaine abusers unlearn old habits associated with cocaine and learn or relearn healthier skills and habits (Carroll, 1998). Cognitive behavior therapy addresses several critical tasks that are essential to successful substance abuse treatment. These include instilling motivation for abstinence, teaching coping skills, and changing reinforcement contingencies necessary, which is necessary, because by the time treatment is sought, many patients or individuals have spent most of their time acquiring, using, and recovering from cocaine to exclusion of other experiences and rewards.

Cognitive behavior therapy is used to identify and reduce habits associated with a drug-using lifestyle by substituting more enduring positive activities and rewards (Carroll, 1998). In addition, CBT fosters management of painful effects by skills training focused on techniques to recognize and cope with urges to use cocaine (Carroll, 1998). Thus, CBT is not only geared to help each individual patient reduce and eliminate substance use while in treatment but also to impart skills that can benefit the patient long after treatment.

Treatment Options

The significance of treating alcohol and drug abuse or dependence cannot be overemphasized. The need for developing treatment programs and approach is more relevant than ever. But it is important to first lay the foundation for a new therapy approach against the background of existing therapy models and interventions. This is why the author took time to review CBT and other models. We will continue to discuss other treatment options that have been documented to work in drug and alcohol treatment below. Therefore, it is critical to first learn about the treatment programs and models presently used in the field of treatment and determine if there is any need to improve the treatment approach to maximize treatment opportunities for individuals.

Community Intervention

This is a community-based action group that provides information training to parents and law enforcement about drug addiction. The group also monitors the community to keep minors away from shops that sell alcohol (Rehnman, Larson, & Andreasson, 2005). According to Rehnman et al., the intervention was shown to be effective, with decreases in sales of alcohol from 73% to 44%.

Social Network Techniques

Social network techniques are based on the presumption that drinking is the result of association. People drink because they see others around them drinking or they had early exposure through their parents or a caretaker. Based on this concept, the treatment targets social networks. The study concluded that drug use is common among individuals with strong social networks where others in their group (parents, friends, coworkers) also use drugs.

State and Federal Treatment

State and Federal government are involved in drug and alcohol treatment prevention by providing funds and treatment programs to support recovery and sobriety. This may also include county behavioral health programs, including drug and alcohol inpatient and outpatient programs. The Federal government spent 3.2 million in the fiscal year of 1998 for alcohol and drug treatment programs (US House of Representatives, Judicial Committee Report, 2000).

Many states have drug and alcohol treatment programs funded by the Substance Abuse and Mental Health Administration. Five percent of state expenditures are spent on prevention, treatment, and research; whereas, the other 95% is spent on incarceration, hospital care, child care, child neglect, poverty, and other social problems that can be associated with alcohol and substance abuse (Heinrich & Hul, 2007). State programs place incompetent individuals to stand trial into state drug and alcohol treatment. Individuals in state and federal custody will receive treatment.

Residential Substance Abuse Treatment: Residential Substance Abuse Treatment (RSAT) for State Prisoners Program assists states and local governments to develop and implement substance abuse treatment programs in state and local correctional and detention facilities (US Department of Justice, 2006). United States Congress established the RSAT program under the Violent Crime Control and Law Enforcement Act of 1994 (Pub. L. No. 103-322, and 1901) (Gonzales, 2005). Residential Substance Abuse Treatment may be used to implement three types of programs for these individuals: residential, jail-based, and aftercare.

Residential programs last for a minimum of six months but no more than twelve months. The program provides residential treatment in separate facilities' apartments or housing units in a facility exclusively for RSAT participants from the general correctional population. The program focuses on substance abuse problems of inmates and requires urinalysis and/or other proven reliable forms of drug and alcohol testing for participants in the custody of the state or local government (US Department of Justice, 2006). Residential treatment may provide opportunities for development of inmates' cognitive, behavioral, social, vocational, and other skills to solve the substance abuse and related problems (US Department of Justice, 2006).

Jail or Local Correctional Facilities Program: Jail treatment may last for three months. The program will attempt to separate the treatment population from the general correction population. Residential substance abuse treatment is generally designed and developed to focus on substance abuse problems of the inmate. The program is generally designed to develop an inmate's cognitive, behavioral, social, vocational, and other skills to solve the substance abuse and related problems (US Department of Justice, 2006).

Mental Health Court/Drug Court Program

Mental health and drug court programs are specialized programs designed to respond to the needs of individuals on divergent programs who otherwise will be serving time instead of treatment. The program normally includes personnel from the courts and mental health staff trained in drug court assessment, proceedings, how to work with court officials, write court reports, and delivery of expert assessment recommendation to help the court determine individuals that will be qualified for divergent programs. My past experience of working in a court has showed me that a court may accept or reject your recommendation, but generally it will not. You must not overdo things and must pay attention to issues and concerns of all parties involved: the district attorney, public defendant or private attorney, the judge, the client, and the government agency you represent as an expert witness. You must work together to achieve what is best for the client to stay clean and sober. It is a fact of life that in some situations some will not respond or comply with the terms of treatment and attend treatment instead of serving time. They will be required to attend weekly treatment: AAA/NA meeting three times a week, drug test, see a therapist, attend recovery outpatient treatment, work with probation and their therapist, comply with the terms of treatment authorized by the court, attend court calendar schedules, complete a treatment program, and graduate from the program. If an individual has disappeared, a warrant will be issued by the judge for their arrest, and if they drug-test positive, they may be reprimanded or have their probation period revoked and then sent to serve all the time on the books for the offense. But courts normally work with individuals to see them succeed.

Aftercare: Aftercare service is generally a coordinated effort between the correction treatment program and other social services and rehabilitation programs, such as education, job training, parole supervision, halfway houses, self-help, and peer group programs (US Department of Justice, 2006). The program may assist inmates in finding community substance abuse treatment facilities on release in conjunction with state and local authorities or organizations (US Department of Justice, 2006).

In-prison Programs: Programs in prison and jails, such as RSAT, serve to educate inmates about substance abuse, including the associated consequences of drug abuse, the abuse cycle, recovery, the relationship of alcohol and drug abuse to problems, and how to work through denial and blaming others for abuse problems (Gonzales, 2005). Offenders learn how to manage anger, stress, and emotions, as well as to resolve conflict and set goals and boundaries. Offenders learn how to develop social skills, communicate, and reinforce positive behavior instead of focusing on negative behaviors. The program may also include a twelve-step program such as Alcoholic Anonymous or Narcotics Anonymous (Gonzales, 2005).

State or Federal alcohol and drug treatment programs use integrated cognitive behavior curriculum concentrated on cognitive restructuring and developing social and problem-solving skills (Gonzales, 2005). The use of the group therapy approach is a key component in treating individuals. Social systems' theory is the underlying behavioral science theory that served to guide group practice (Taubman, 2006). Group treatment depends on utilizing different psychological theories as guiding principles in pre-arranging the group, starting the group, and working with the group through implementation and facilitation.

Because this study is about describing qualitative therapy group practice and analysis, it is recommended we first lay the theoretical foundation of as to why the author reasons that qualitative therapy holds a good prospect for improving clinical practice in addiction treatment because of its rich potential for exploring phenomena unknown and to learn about the phenomena for the purpose of grasping the problem in real experience directly through interviews and indirectly through data analysis. This potential offers a wide opportunity for taking addiction treatment to another level with the use of scientific analysis steps for understanding the nature, categories, patterns, and risk levels associated with pretreatment addiction relapse triggers. It is not just enough to talk about triggers, but you have to show and represent what they are. Qualitative therapy and analysis offers this rare possibility hardly used in addiction therapy before this report. In the next chapter, chapter three, we will discuss the theoretical support for qualitative therapy.

CHAPTER THREE

Qualitative Therapy Model

Qualitative therapy was developed by the author with the assumption that all symptoms associated with a disease start, develop, and progress in a horizontal context before they are diagnosed and treatment starts. More often than not, in medical practice, the horizontal context may not be a part or focus of the treatment but that of symptom reduction and in addiction, modification of behavior, thoughts, and feelings. Horizontal context is the practical setting of all disease and addiction and should not be ignored or allowed to pass by unnoticed. It is because disease or addiction develops in a real horizontal relationship and later shows itself in symptoms and in psychiatric or psychological medicine in thoughts, feelings, and behavior. Horizontal context has very concrete terms and properties and includes poor diet, stress, social triggers for emotional distress, lack of resources to maintain a healthy lifestyle and maintenance, relationship problems, lack of physical exercise, undiagnosed and untreated symptoms and trigger response, prenatal undiagnosed genetic problems in parents that are passed on to their children, etc. Each of these will manifest themselves in a disease process. Unless the horizontal context of a disease becomes the focus of treatment as well as that of the symptoms, conditions will not improve because the patient or addicts will return after being discharged to the same horizontal context that may have contributed to a symptom or will continue to worsen in condition once a disease or condition has been diagnosed. Therefore, developing a treatment process to access general information in the horizontal context is as critical as finding symptoms and the treatment. The author here describes the process that may be used to learn about the horizontal context to include the treatment's goals and objectives.

This study was designed to describe qualitative therapy group model practice. But first, we will discuss the theoretical foundation for qualitative therapy, drawing from the application of qualitative research theories and principles wherever applicable.

In this chapter, the author has outlined the theory of qualitative therapy model and group practice developed as part of his regular Education for Recovery in Addiction (ERA) group treatment, called *Qualitative Therapy*, for identifying pretreatment relapse triggers.

Qualitative (Q) therapy model includes finding out what people think, feel, and do before and during the time they relapsed. In the qualitative therapy model, addiction is viewed as a phenomena rather than a disease. Therapy becomes a vehicle for understanding the phenomena or problem for descriptive understanding by the therapist in his or her own filters and information on the topic. This is the striking difference between qualitative therapy and all existing models of therapy. The assumption is that individual experiences are generally unknown to others and the therapist and vary greatly; therefore, these experiences need to be captured for a better understanding of the accurate relapse issues and challenges observed or unobserved. Thus, the therapist develops his personal observations, reflects on his personal weekly notes, flip charts, observation, personal reflection, and theories for understanding the phenomena and in planning intervention for constructing a clean and sober life. Many times, drug and alcohol treatment are designed to fit a general model or are tailored to fit an existing model. The present existing drug and alcohol treatment models may be designed to focus on a specific outcome, including cognitive behavior modification, than identifying and working with pretreatment relapse triggers. No doubt CBT and other existing models have been documented to be effective for what they were designed to achieve. Therefore, constructing a clean and sober life will first require an understanding of the phenomena or the relapse problem.

Qualitative therapy was developed with the goal in mind to first understand the phenomena or relapse problem by identifying the pretreatment addiction relapse triggers, teach appropriate trigger responses necessary for relapse prevention, and construct a clean and sober life with awareness of exposure to trigger risk. This goal was accomplished by the author by maintaining a specific focus on: (a) motivation for drug and alcohol use; (b) relapse triggers; (c) problems associated with drug use; (d) chemical effects of alcohol and drug use; (e) financial cost; (f) community relapse problems; (g) crime and arrest; and (h) staying clean and sober. The fact is that individuals with a frequent relapse history may have a problem in understanding what a clean and sober life is because they never lived it or they have had only a brief experience of a clean and sober life. This becomes a major issue in treatment: how to prepare an individual for living a clean and sober life when he or she has difficulty staying clean and sober. Many individuals are prepared to abstain from or stop using drugs, but they are not prepared to first understand the phenomena of the relapse problem because it will require researching the phenomena than assessing the phenomena for treatment. Researching the phenomena will require understanding steps of descriptive research for correct application in group treatment or process for identifying the problem and the intricacies and complexities.

One reason for this problem is that treatment is focused on the person than the person in the community facing barrages of relapse trigger problems he or she has failed to take on or is too scared to walk back into. This mistake continues even as I am writing this book because some treatment programs stop at changing the behavior or thought process and not on taking on the individual in the community.

If a client is discharged without a clear understanding of the pretreatment relapse triggers that contributed to his or her relapsed behavior and trouble with the law, they will return to the life they were living before they relapsed, were arrested, and then sent for treatment. This is the life they knew. An effective treatment program should go beyond learning how to stop using drugs; it should be about bringing about behavioral changes, thoughts, or feelings and reconstructing the life of an addict. The steps to reconstruct patterns of pretreatment addiction relapse trigger have not been developed. If and when they are developed, they should at least offer a prospect and possibility for use in identifying pretreatment relapse triggers, relapse behavior, and challenges. But first, what is urgently needed is a psycho-educational group therapy model for process and identification of pretreatment addiction relapse trigger. The author will discuss how he discovered it and the most effective way it can be done from his experience of developing and using the qualitative group therapy approach adapted from qualitative therapy theory and principles.

Qualitative Group Therapeutic Relationships

The author developed a qualitative or Q therapy after he discovered that qualitative therapy principles can be used and adapted into a psycho-educational therapy for understanding pretreatment addiction relapse triggers. The author studied a broad range of present therapy practices, including research method, searching for the best approach with a broad range of scientific potential, including analysis of pretreatment addiction relapse triggers. In qualitative group therapy, the focus is on developing a relationship between the individual and the therapist, which will provide an environment conducive to exploring pretreatment addiction relapse triggers in the environment or phenomena. The author has developed and used the following techniques below:

Qualitative Group Techniques

1. Focused on group pretreatment addiction and unobserved experiences by asking many questions, one per day, in group sessions for twelve weeks.
2. Wrote the questions on the board or flip chart prior to the commencement of the group, asked the questions in the group, and waited for the group response.
3. Focused on the relationships: how the group or individuals described their experiences, how they felt about their addiction and associated problems, and how they described the interactions in addiction. The author wrote down the triggers, risks, and physical, social, and chemical impacts of the use of substances described by the group, and noted the pretreatment relapse trigger characteristics and patterns emerging from the group.
4. Supported the group and encouraged them to share their experiences.

5. Validated the experience of the group by writing their responses on the board, reviewing them with the group before the group was dismissed, and reviewing them again the following week.

6. The generated data were stored as general educational information for understanding pretreatment addiction relapse triggers, ongoing group facilitation, discussion, comparison of responses, and experience.

Qualitative Group Task

According to the author, his task during group sessions was to ask questions and document what he saw and heard, in his own words. Answers to questions were not only documented in terms of textual detail but also in the internal act of consideration, experiencing, as such, rhythm and relationship between the phenomena and self (Moustakas, 1994). The second task is deciding how to use the information for topic notes and intervention development. But group process is not enough without analysis for in-depth analysis of the trigger leading to finding out why people use drugs, bringing together all information available on the topic for analysis. This is the main purpose of this study analysis. But before we get to that, we need to learn about qualitative group plan and application.

Qualitative Group Plan and Application

To facilitate qualitative group therapy or Q therapy, the author has developed a plan for starting group sessions, normally twelve in one segment for twelve weeks. The plan must have the following: (a) date; (b) number of participants (male or female); (c) group topic; (d) group question; (e) group answer or response written down; and (f) material and tools (pencil, paper, flip charts, markers, notepad, and word processor) for the group process.

Group Guidelines: For each session, the author as a therapist at the time welcomed the group, discussed group rules and breaks, and announced the topic to be covered in the group.

Group Process Session: Twelve questions were developed for twelve group sessions. The author designed the questions to explore the topic: (a) a general open-ended question; and (b) a written question for individuals to answer on an answer sheet and return.

Group sessions' questions were written on a flip chart. The group was invited to respond to the question and share their experiences about addiction in the community. A volunteer from among the group wrote the responses on the flip chart. The researcher recorded the responses in a notepad, to be later transcribed by typing them into his general note on the topic. During the group session, the author discussed the answers with the group and gave the group time to react, and he also contributed any theoretical information related to the topic. The author reviewed the answers with the group to summarize key points before the end of each group session and the beginning of each new session. The author also compared responses to the same question from other sources, including research, group responses, summary, and review. In this way, the author guarantees consistent and new information on the topic of triggers.

Before the end of a session, the author: (a) summarized key points; (b) announced the next group session; (c) gave an assignment to be completed by the next session; (d) thanked; and (d) dismissed the group. The author summarized his recollection of key points and added that to his topic notes on the subject for summary and reviews, and that way he maintained up-to-date information on the topic of trigger not found anywhere else that informed his understanding of pretreatment addiction relapse trigger. Notes are of key importance other than chart notes to study for understanding a phenomenon like addiction relapse trigger. Notes offer a wide range of possibilities for study, summary, reviews, and updating new information on a topic, where less is known about pretreatment addiction relapse triggers among forensic population in the Inland Empire in California. This is the unique contribution of this study when we get to the analysis section of this study for understanding the categories, patterns, and risk levels of pretreatment addiction relapse trigger.

Ratcliff (n.d.) stated that handwritten notes can be typed. In addition, during the typing process, the therapist may recall some details that were not written down during the interview. Impressions, feelings, self-reflections, and memories should be recorded in notes. Types of notes that the therapist can take are shown in Table 2. General notes on a topic on which there is very little information on a population in the Inland Empire is of key importance for working with forensic population. General topic notes on a phenomenon are different from individual chart notes because they are general and topic oriented than individual tailored. They offer collective understanding of a topic or phenomena on which very little is known, exists, or is gathered, and they can be studied for cumulative understanding and treatment development. It is from notes that you develop an expertise on a given topic or phenomena about which very little information exists and less is available to go on because no one has spent time other than giving therapy group or individuals to develop notes on the phenomena for understanding a problem most are willing to treat than to study and then treat.

This longitudinal gathering of note or data allows the researcher the latitude to compare different groups' answers for the purpose of developing an understanding of pretreatment relapse triggers.

Table 2
Note Types

Note type	Description
Field notes	Running accounts of what happened during the interview, or transcripts of video or audiotape.
Theoretical notes	Accounts that include emergent trends; hypotheses, which would have to be tested; guesses; and hunches.
Methodology notes	Descriptions of methods used; reason for taking notes. These are useful for review.

The notes are not in or part of the personal identifiable medical record files of individuals. They are general notes on addiction and pretreatment relapse triggers. Therefore, there are no specific or individual references or names of individuals who participated in the groups within the data. Anonymity of participants was maintained, and there is no possibility of identifying a group member or individual problem or response. The data, therefore, reflect the researcher reflection, new insight, theories, and flip chart information on triggers.

CHAPTER FOUR

Method and Design

In this chapter, we will learn about the steps for data analysis which are of key importance for understanding horizontal addiction categories, patterns, risks, and challenges.

We have now approached the good part of this study, which is the purpose for which this study was proposed: developing research analysis steps using a scientific method for analysis of notes on pretreatment addiction relapse trigger affecting Inland Empire forensic population in California. Unless we develop the steps for analysis, we will not be able to complete the analysis for understanding pretreatment addiction relapse triggers in the Inland Empire forensic population. Inland Empire addiction problems present one of the most difficult challenges in addiction treatment because of the population and diversity groups affected by addiction disease that has been growing. Therefore, finding a way of studying about it using a scientific process will offer rare possibilities not available anywhere. We are familiar with research methods, both quantitative and qualitative methods, and researchers use them every day. The author discovered that the same research method can be used to develop qualitative therapy for group processes and also for the analysis proposed in this study. This will change the way we use qualitative research from now on. Qualitative research principles offer long-time effect on how we adapt it in qualitative group therapy and for analysis of trigger categories, patterns, and risk levels, an approach not used before but that which has potential to become the therapy for the twenty-first century addiction treatment. The author has realized that a lot is thrown around about triggers and a lot of individuals are behind bars or in treatment or have their life ruined over addiction problems; therefore, we must come up with either tools or steps to analyze triggers instead of just talking about them. We must be able to show through the use of scientific analysis the impact of different triggers on individuals for developing treatment that will minimize ongoing relapse or recidivism. Equally important is to find out first what the relapse triggers are contributing to the behavior, what kind of triggers people battling with the disease of addiction are confronting, the nature of the triggers, kind of triggers, and the volume a person may experience before they relapse, how strong they are, why and the risk and level of risk a person battling with addiction may be experiencing a time or over a time, and the impact of the drug or alcohol and the trigger on a person's mental health, psychology, physical health, mood, and behavior.

We do not know the answers just yet, but finding a way of knowing is of key importance in planning a treatment for recovery. This is why, this chapter is very important.

Further, an understanding of pretreatment addiction relapse trigger will require an analysis for a better understanding of pretreatment addiction relapse trigger categories, patterns, and risk levels. Also, analysis will be necessary and equally important for developing treatment options and targets because it is not just enough to diagnose if a person is an addict without showing it and representing it backed by scientific means showing the categories, patterns, and risk levels. Gone are the days when we treated and there was no data to show how we arrived at what we were treating and what you think you are treating to prevent relapse.

According to Young et al. (2001), in the general population, the rate of recidivism is 86% two years after treatment, with the majority of the relapses occurring within six months of treatment. If we want to help save people affected by the disease of addiction, we must have tools and steps to explain how to organize data that will help us learn and understand pretreatment relapse triggers and problems.

In this chapter, you will learn about steps how to organize your observation, topic notes, curriculum notes, theories, and flip chart information for analysis using qualitative research methods and data analysis techniques developed in this study. Data analysis involves the coding of the data. This kind of analysis involves a description of what the researcher wants to know about a problem or topic and how the findings are coded to learn about the various aspects of the problem or topic. This process is generally referred to as qualitative archival analysis. The purpose of an analysis is to provide valuable generalized information to illustrate a topic, issue, or concern dedicated toward the study of a close relationship of triggers and relapse behaviors for policy and treatment purpose. The analysis will become a most valuable skill for enhanced understanding and presentation of pretreatment addiction relapse triggers. It will change from now on as to how we identify and present, using scientific means, triggers for developing drug and alcohol relapse prevention treatment intervention and for supporting our claims and bills to receive reimbursement for treatment developed and administered. The steps presented here are free, and the author does not charge for it; it is a gift to drug and alcohol treatment communities.

Before you get to analyze anything, you got to have developed the questions you have in mind that you want to find answers for. Each question should guide the analysis of the data, in this case topic notes, on pretreatment addiction relapse trigger. In the next paragraph that follows, you will see a list of questions developed by the author to guide the analysis until it is completed.

Analysis Questions

Each question guided the study. The author generated the questions for analysis below:

1. According to the data, what will the data tell us about the nature of addiction trigger?
2. What are the causes, patterns, and categories of pretreatment addiction relapse triggers found in the data?
3. Based on the study, what is the most effective way of treating pretreatment addiction relapse triggers and relapse risk?
4. How does the qualitative therapy approach for Education for Recovery and Addiction, ERA, which targets the revealed risks

and relapse triggers, contribute current research understanding of pretreatment addiction relapse triggers and prompt recommendation for relapse prevention and discharge readiness before a patient is released into the same or similar community or neighborhood he or she relapsed and was arrested from?

These questions provide the direction to take in analyzing the data for understanding pretreatment addiction relapse triggers. Take it from me, what we do not understand is that there is a close connection between relapse behavior and triggers; we need to understand the causes, patterns, categories, and risks posed by triggers by using a scientific approach used in this study. It is the new way forward because we can demonstrate what triggers we identify with a specific population or group or from the data we analyzed. This is important to show and back what we are treating and how we plan to treat whether we go after the thought, feelings, behavior, or the triggers fortifying patients with knowledge and skills to respond to triggers in their environment. Unfortunately, no two triggers are the same or carry the same risk for all groups. This is what we may soon learn after the result of the analysis is presented.

Method and Design

The author in an attempt to find answers to the research questions and other relevant questions utilized a qualitative, grounded theory, designed to examine the pretreatment addiction relapse triggers notes utilized in the analysis as well as the efficacy of the use of qualitative measures to uncover and evaluate relapse triggers for the development of prevention programs. In contrast, quantitative approaches are most often used when the variables of the problem are clearly defined (Creswell, 2005).

In the case of this study, where the data consisted of the lived experiences, beliefs, and truths of individuals, there are no hypotheses that can be pre-set with regard to individual specific relapse triggers; rather, theory was formed and supported by the identified themes that emerged from the data. The following sections include discussions of the research method, the research design, and the appropriateness of the design for the study.

Research Method

Creswell (2005) states, "Qualitative research is suited for researching problems in which the problem variables are unknown and need to be explored" (p. 45). The grounded theory was selected for this study because the research served to explore the lived experiences and perceptions of participants from the data, rather than to quantify variable relationships. Qualitative studies maintain a focus on the participant's perspective and the personal meaning held by the participant (Creswell, 2005).

The qualitative grounded theory method also provides flexibility in exploring a subject while allowing an in-depth investigation, potentially leading to the development of a new observation and the opportunity for further exploration of a study's prevalence, predictors, and sequence in other studies (Yoshikawa, Weisner, Kalil, & Way, 2008). Qualitative methods are inquiry-based, enabling the exploration of an occurrence through questions, narrative descriptions, and analysis of emerging themes (Creswell, 2005). Qualitative methods provide a representation of the specific focus of the study, based on the interpretation of lived experiences of the group therapy participants (Creswell, 2005; Neuman, 2003).

Patton (2002) explained why the qualitative approach may be useful for analyzing pretreatment trigger experiences. He stated that the issue is not whether research data is more desirable, valid, or meaningful than self-reported data; the fact is that therapists cannot observe what individuals have done in their pretreatment addiction phase and lifestyle before coming for help or treatment. It is important to learn what the addicts' thoughts and behavior were before and after they became addicted.

In response to this need, a study was developed to analyze the ERA data for understanding pretreatment addiction relapse triggers, in an effort to minimize them. The researcher employed a qualitative grounded theory design to study the phenomenon by analyzing data collected from 2008 to 2009 in groups that explored pretreatment addiction relapse triggers.

Research Design

The qualitative grounded theory design is a qualitative method used to generate a theory based on the information collected from the participants; as such, the purpose of grounded theory design is to enable research in which theory can emerge from data-driven methods (Creswell, 2007; Glaser & Strauss, 2009). Glaser and Strauss posited that data collection could lead to a theory that can be used later in practical application. The grounded theory design is useful for explaining the experiences, events, activities, actions, and intentions of research study participants (Creswell, 2005; Glaser & Strauss, 2009). In addition, the grounded theory design provides a systematic approach that can be followed to provide relevant and academically sound results (Hunter, Hari, Egbu, & Kelly, 2005).

Creswell (2005), states, "Grounded theory design is a systematic, qualitative procedure used to generate a theory that explains at a broad conceptual level, process, action, or interaction about a substantive topic" (p. 396). In the case of this study, the conceptual theory that was generated serves to explain the complexities of relapse triggers among the forensic individuals with drug—and alcohol-related problems and the interaction of the use of qualitative methods with the development of successful relapse prevention techniques for these individuals. The grounded theory design was appropriate for this study because it adds a predictive and inductive aspect that takes the experiences of the research participants and moves the experiences to predictive tools (Creswell, 2005; Hunter et al., 2005).

Therefore, a qualitative grounded theory design was used in the analysis by the author to analyze the questions and answers raised in the study. In addition, the researcher developed a list of all questions asked and the responses given. The steps the researcher employed included looking at each question and searching the data for the answer through content analysis.

Krippendorff (2004) indicated that content analysis is an empirically grounded theory. In addition, content analysis transcends traditional notions of symbols, content, and intent. Empirical evidence is gathered such that an exploratory approach is used during the process of the study, while the resulting content analysis produces predictive or inferential intent.

Content analysis requires examination of multiple document data sources to develop a thorough comprehension of the various textual data researched (Neuendorf, 2002). Content analysis can be used to decipher certain concepts present in texts or written documents (Neuendorf, 2002). The purpose of determining themes and concepts within documentation or texts is to enable the investigator to quantify and analyze the data such that inferences about the written text can be made. Content analysis was used in conjunction with the grounded theory to provide the results of the study.

Data and Sampling

The study examined ex-post facto data in the form of observations and topic notes generated during the application of qualitative group process in an Education for Recovery in Addiction group as topic notes on triggers used in general group summaries, weekly reviews, and follow-up three years prior to the present study and analysis. The data will became an invaluable (Patton, 2002) information for analyzing and understanding pretreatment addiction relapse trigger among forensic individuals in the Inland Empire and for comparing information on trigger presented in the literature review in chapter two. How important is data sampling for addiction treatment? My general impression is that we are living in the image of information technology when talking about information or access can mean creating a new understanding of a disease, in this case—addiction. We use information every day in health system for billing and treatment. But we need to go a step further where information is used for study and analysis, to figure out a health phenomenon, issues, or problems that can put us one step ahead of a relapse or relapse trigger and we can help minimize the risk. With data analysis, a clinician will be able to analyze and figure out categories, patterns, and risk levels of a vector or trigger to enhance treatment and also billing. Because, as you will find out, the instrument used in the analysis study to write this book has a lot of potential for helping us learn about triggers among forensic population, with an eye to understand the history, patterns, categories, and risk levels of pretreatment addiction relapse trigger. Addiction analysis is a new field in addiction, and I am sure with this start, it will grow and more new tools will be developed to show real-time analysis of pretreatment addiction relapse triggers for billing purpose and for treatment and intervention development.

The archival sources included data from flip chart, ERA group curriculum notes, and intranet information obtained from previous ERA groups in which the qualitative method was utilized for facilitating the group process on addiction. Each group met for two twelve-week sessions.

In this study, the sample for analysis, therefore, comprised a purposeful sample. Purposeful sampling is a non-probabilistic sampling method in which the researcher selects particular research locations and participants to increase the probability that they will be able to provide the information necessary to answer the research questions of the study (Creswell, 2005). Selecting qualitative samples focuses on a collection of participants who provide specific narratives to clarify and deepen the exploration of the study (Neuman, 2003). Since this study only included analysis of archival data, it did not involve a direct contact with individuals.

Qualitative research normally involves small sample sizes of participants, in contrast to quantitative research, which typically involves larger sample sizes (Creswell, 2005). Although Creswell (2005) and Polkinghorne (2005) recommended that the size of a qualitative sample should range from—one to twenty-five participants and—five to twenty-five participants respectively, Patton (2002) stated that there are no specific rules for sample size, and he stated, "Sample size depends on what you want to know, the purpose of the inquiry, what's at stake, what will be useful, what will have credibility, and what can be done with available time and resources" (p. 244). In this study, the sample size are documented notes and flip charts, etc., selected for analysis.

Population

The analysis does not involve direct contact with individuals but only archival data from flip charts, group response to questions and answers written on flip charts, therapist group comments, insights, explanation, and intranet information compiled and typed by the researcher in the ERA qualitative group curriculum used by the researcher for end-of-group reviews and weekly reviews and follow-up on key points.

Confidentiality is an important responsibility of the researcher when conducting research. Confidentiality is the process of holding participants' personal information in confidence without disclosure to the public (Neuman, 2003). The study involved no individual identifiable data such as name, address, employer, relatives' names, date of birth, telephone number, e-mail address, Social Security number, account information, voiceprint, fingerprint, photos, personal chart information, or any other characteristic that may identify an individual in group treatment. All information gathered in the curriculum notes remained anonymous and general.

Instrumentation

The instruments in this study included a set of open-ended questions developed by the researcher to reflect the pattern in the curriculum notes.

Questions played a key role in analysis coding. Coding often involves a series of questions. In this study, the data for the analysis have already been collected. Therefore, the questions to which participants responded during the group process guided the coding and analysis (Braun & Clarke, 2006).

Within a grounded theory framework, the essence of what the author documented in the notes on trigger from groups over several years was extracted and analyzed in order to determine the nature and characteristics of pretreatment addiction triggers. In addition, a theory was generated that demonstrates the capability of the qualitative approach in producing prevention strategies targeted at relapse triggers.

The data was gathered and developed and used in the study for analysis in the form of typed notes (Ratcliff, n.d.) made for group process, review, follow-up, and for understanding the vector of trigger and relapse behavior among forensic individuals. All group notes used in the study and analysis were preserved; they are cover data obtained from different groups on addiction.

The archival data included descriptive accounts of what happened during group treatment, theoretical information that included emergent trends, hypotheses, guesses, hunches, methodology, and descriptions of methods used during the group process. The data also included information about the group's pretreatment addiction trigger experiences and responses.

The note was used in the study as a unit of analysis. What was interesting was that no two groups have the same responses on pretreatment addiction relapse triggers. One group's response recorded was different from the other group's response, providing a variety of responses to the same question asked and processed during a qualitative group session over several years. The notes have cumulative information on pretreatment addiction relapse trigger, and that is why the notes are useful for analysis and for understanding the nature of pretreatment addiction relapse trigger among forensic individuals. But the information does not substitute for other research that has been done or medical consultation on addiction problem.

Steps

A qualitative grounded theory approach was employed in the analysis, along with content analysis techniques. To conduct a content analysis on the text obtained for this research, the data were coded into manageable categories on a variety of levels (Neuendorf, 2002). It included breaking the textual data down into key components, words, sentences, or themes. These themes or key components were then examined using relational analysis to determine whether there were any relationships among the responses of the subjects.

Leedy and Ormrod (2005) stated, "A grounded theory study uses a prescribed set of procedures for analysing data and constructing a theoretical model from them" (p. 140). Glaser and Strauss (2009) outlined a four-step process for data analysis in grounded theory designs. The first step of the grounded theory process described by Glaser and Strauss (2009) involves developing the codes to be used in the analysis. This allowed the researcher to collate the types of information required to answer the central research questions of the study.

The second step of the process, as outlined by Glaser and Strauss (2009), requires the collection of the different concepts determined by the codes used in the first stage of the process; as such, the researcher grouped together the codes that have similar content.

The third step of the grounded theory process calls for the categorization of the concepts that were grouped in the previous step. This allowed the author-researcher to determine the different aspects of the risks and triggers for the participants, the common psychological and sociological influences, and the perceived efficacy of the qualitative group approach.

The fourth step in the grounded theory process for the study was to define the theory that was determined. Once the theory was established, the researcher was then able to explain the phenomenon as perceived by the group participants.

Patton (2002) listed the steps involved in data analysis as follows: (a) conceptual ordering; (b) theorizing; (c) microanalysis; (d) theoretical sampling; (e) theoretical saturation; (f) range of variability; (g) open coding; (h) axial coding; and (i) relationship statement (explanation of the what, why, where, and how of the phenomenon, or the problem study in relation to the responses given).

The open-ended question response data were coded to identify open coding categories (Creswell, 2005). Open coding categories were created with the assistance of NVivo8® qualitative coding software, which assisted in the coding, categorization, and frequency determination of categories within the transcribed textual data, allowing for the transformation of the data into theoretical groups that can in turn be used to build constructs and theory. Coding software is suggested as a helpful tool for coding grounded theory data because the software helps to organize and create meaning within the complex data collected during a grounded theory research project (Hunter et al., 2005). The open coding categories assisted in determining the selective coding categories. The selective coding categories were related to the central theme, which emerged from the findings related to resistance. From this point, a narrative was created to describe the interrelationships of the selected coding, and finally, the consequences of the core phenomenon of an axial diagram. Once the data have been collected and coded and themes have emerged, the research report was created, which was validated both internally and externally.

The future use of software in addiction analysis has begun. This research has paved the way forward that it is not just enough to talk about triggers, it must be clinically represented by the use of software not only for billing but also for figuring out and revealing and developing an understanding of the history of the triggers present in a group: the categories, patterns, and risk levels for developing appropriate responses to minimize ongoing repeated relapse. This is just the beginning; we will soon be training therapists across the country on how to run qualitative group therapy and how to analyze history of pretreatment addiction relapse trigger for treatment planning, trigger risk identification, categorization, patterns, and minimizing the risk for relapse before it happens. The ball has begun rolling. We shall see how this was done in this study in chapter five where the analysis result is presented.

Assumptions

The theoretical assumption used for integrating qualitative phenomenological methods into the ERA group therapy was that individuals are affected by unknown and unobserved experiences that dominate their lives. The unknown in the mind of the individual in treatment holds the cues or triggers that can affect the progress of drug use or relapse. Thus, it is very important to tap into that unknown experience base prior to reaching out into existing evidence-based descriptive information. Individuals, therapists, and loved ones should first avail themselves of the unknown and unobserved reality of relapse experience available from the group or individual, in order to be effective in processing and planning intervention.

It was assumed that knowing this experience-based information helps the clinician and the group to understand realities from a descriptive phenomenon, identify and reduce conflict, and increase cooperation and interest through meaning, recognition, and exchange. The last assumption the author-researcher had was that if we could use an existing tool or software and analyze the notes, it could reveal an understanding of the history of pretreatment addiction triggers within the notes or data, with an eye to understanding the phenomena of relapse among forensic individuals for treatment development.

Validity and Reliability

Validity is based on determining whether the findings are accurate from the standpoint of the researcher, the participant, or the readers of an account, whereas reliability evidences that the approach can be consistent across different researchers and projects (Creswell, 2005, 2007). The validity and reliability of the study were enhanced by incorporating the process of *member checking* (Creswell, 2005). According to the information in the notes or data, each group had time to review the past and went over the summary of points at the beginning and end of each group that went on for years. During the summary, groups, along with the group leaders, reviewed and checked the recorded data on the flip chart or blackboard to ensure that data accurately described and validated key points. Also, using member checking, the group in a sense ensured that the group participants felt the descriptions in the review before the start of a new topic, and the end of the group summary was accurate, complete, and true to the different groups' relapse experience to be compiled in general the information notes on pretreatment addiction relapse trigger used in this study and analysis.

Yin (1994) suggested reporting a detailed protocol for data collection so that the procedure of a qualitative study might be replicated in another setting. Therefore, in order to ensure reliability of the study, the collection of data followed the procedure described in the previous data analysis section. Qualitative validity was also improved using NVivo 8® qualitative analysis software to aid in the coding and categorization of the data. We can be certain that the curriculum notes used in the study for analysis are based on observation and documentation of a process involving group reviews and sharing of information in which individuals within each group had time and opportunity to respond to answers.

Data Analysis

The study utilized ex-post facto data in the form of observations and field notes generated from use of qualitative open-ended questioning during two Educations for Recovery from in Addiction (ERA) groups led by a facilitator. The group sits in numbers of about twenty-four to forty individuals, male and female, representing White, Black, Asian, Native American, Hispanics, and other South American population. Notes about the process were typed and added daily to other general notes on pretreatment addiction relapse triggers used in weekly reviews and summary for twelve weeks per session four sessions per year for several years.

The author used these compiled notes to analyze pretreatment addiction relapse triggers for understanding historical and present risks posed by these triggers to a group or individuals. The notes were also analyzed for common psychological and sociological influences, as well as perceived efficacy of qualitative group therapy application. The analysis process also included content analysis on the data or text for understanding problems associated with relapse triggers. The data was coded into manageable categories, which included breaking the textual data down into key components, words, sentences, or themes. These themes or key components were then examined using relational analysis to determine whether there are any relationships between the responses of the subjects. The final stage in the grounded theory process was to define the theory that was determined. Data analysis is going to be the next big move in health care not only for billing purpose but also because of the value general notes outside of patients' chart notes offers for understanding and developing treatment for a phenomena common to a group. I often say to a friend note on a giving problem will become the next textbook assignment for understanding a problem outside of individual chart notes. When notes are analyzed from general observation using scientific methods and software, they give more in-depth analysis of a problem demonstrated in this study for better understanding of the problem and for comparison and contrast. In the next chapter, chapter five, we will see the analysis result from the data used in the analysis. Qualitative analysis is always guided by questions about unknowns unlike quantitative method where the hypothesis or what is already known will be tested. In this study, we do not have any hypothesis to test or any information about the question or questions we want to learn about until the analysis is completed; only then can we develop a theoretical framework or understanding about what is driving the demand for drug use in USA. But before we go to the analysis result and report in the next chapter, let us review again the questions we want to have answered. This will help us understand the findings of the analysis report. The questions are as follows:

1. According to the data, what will the data tell the author/researcher about the nature of addiction trigger among forensic population?

2. What are the causes, patterns, and categories of pretreatment addiction relapse triggers experienced by forensic individuals found in the data proposed for analysis?

3. Based on the study, what is the most effective way of treating pretreatment addiction relapse triggers?

4. How does qualitative group therapy approach in Education for Recovery in Addiction, which targets the revealed risks and pretreatment relapse triggers contributing to the current research understanding of pretreatment addiction relapse prevention and discharge readiness before a client is released and discharged to the same or similar community or neighborhood he or she relapsed and was arrested from?

CHAPTER FIVE

What Is Driving Demand?
For Drug Use

Results

The author cannot stop stressing the importance of analytic science in drug and alcohol treatment. The science is very important for identifying categories, patterns, and risks associated with pretreatment addiction relapse trigger. Also, the science of this will help a clinician represent vividly the kind of triggers affecting a specific population or group and incorporate that information in treatment development and intervention. Trigger analysis can also be used for trigger response training for minimizing frequent relapse, particularly in addiction cases where there has been a similar trigger exposure over months and years.

Why is trigger analysis and its results important in drug and alcohol treatment? Without analysis, you really cannot describe the category, patterns, and risks associated with triggers and relapse behavior. Also, you cannot start planning treatment if you have no way of finding the nature of triggers affecting a group, population, or individual. Triggers can also be good for billing purposes because you will be able to show what triggers you have identified contributing to relapse behavior and how you plan to minimize the impact. Trigger identification and analysis will be the next way to go in drug and alcohol treatment because it will contribute big-time to understanding relapse behavior. A study by Terrence T. Gorster and Merlene Miller in 1982 identified a set of warning signs or steps that typically will lead up to a relapse as follows: change in attitude; elevated stress; reactivation of denial; recurring withdrawal symptoms, like behavior change, social breakdown; loss structure; loss of judgment; loss of control; and loss of option. While this may apply in that study in 1982, what will this study identify and describe what a trigger is and what will be the difference in terms of new methods, information, and contribution to forensic psychology of addiction and prevention?

According to Young et al. (2001), in the general population, the rate of recidivism is 86% two years after treatment, with the majority of the relapses occurring within six months of treatment. What is driving the demand for drug use in America and what can be done about it to save life? The author responded to this question in this chapter. Let us read what the author found from his data analysis.

Why Use Drugs?

The first thematic category revealed from the data analysis was related to the responses given with regard to why people want to use drugs. The data contained information and reasons about why people want to use drugs or keep using drugs and/or perceptions of other reasons that others may use drugs. The results indicate a predominance of three areas: emotional reasons, escape, and addiction. Table 2 illustrates the five overall categories of reasons for using drugs and the frequency of these types of elements mentioned by participants. The key here is often the expectation of what the perceiver thinks or feels about what the desired effect they will experience during or after they self-administered the drugs. It is important as the author compares that with the real experience after the drugs have been administered or ingested. The key here is learning about addiction relapse triggers and how triggers drive or influence relapse behavior and the complexities and challenges and what we should do after we learn about the triggers and the implication for recovery, planning relapse behavior, and putting in place steps to minimize triggers from influencing a relapse behavior that will trigger other unforeseen behaviors and problems.

Then and only then can we say we have a scientific data that shows what direction we focus our resources to help individuals or groups battling with addiction. The rule is that no trigger should be left unexplored or dismissed as too small so as to wreak havoc when it comes to human behavior. From experience, people overwhelmed with domestic challenges may relapse and use the most negative coping skills that may put them in trouble with the law.

Table 3

Perceptions of Why People Want to Use Drugs

	Group 1	Group 2	Total No. of Responses
Emotional reasons	**23**	**24**	**47**
Depression	2	3	5
Emotional problems (sadness, anger, disappointment)	1	5	6
Suicidal or other bad thoughts		2	2
To feel good or happier	11	6	17
Boredom	5	2	7
Low self-esteem		1	1
Lack of hope/apathy		2	2
Uninhibited		2	2
Satisfy curiosity	3	1	4
Stupidity	1		1
To escape various problems	**15**	**10**	**25**
To escape problems in general	3	7	10
Family problems	1	1	2
Losing a child or friend	2	1	3
For self-medicating		1	1
To relax	5		5
Stress	4		4

Addiction-related reasons	**13**	**9**	**22**
Addiction	3	2	5
To get high	5	2	7
Desire/craving	1	1	2
Habit		2	2
Like it	4	2	6
Physical reasons	**1**	**5**	**6**
More energy	1	1	2
Weight loss		1	1
Appetite		1	1
Sexual stimulation		1	1
Health		1	1
Social reasons	**4**	**8**	**12**
Relationships		1	1
To make money	1	3	4
Fun	2		2
Free time		1	1
Dramatics		1	1
Prison	1	1	2
Want to be famous		1	1

The first types of responses are (as noted in Table 1) elements that could be classified as emotional responses. These included the following elements found in the data: depression, emotional problems such as extreme sadness, anger, or disappointment, suicidal thoughts/ bad thoughts, to feel good/happier, boredom, low self-esteem, lack of hope/apathy, uninhibited, satisfy curiosity, and stupidity. Of these elements, the desire to feel good or happier was mentioned most often. Overall, emotional reasons for using drugs was the most commonly cited reason and accounted for forty-seven mentions by participants in both groups, with twenty-three elements coming from group one and twenty-four of these elements stemming from data from group two, demonstrating a similarity of responses between groups. The variety of responses given in Table 1 demonstrate perceptions of the reasons for using drugs and illustrate the diversity of reasons for which the initiation of drug use ensues. This is critical to understanding the elements that also contribute to relapse.

The second and third types of responses found include: (a) use as an escape mechanism; and (b) addiction. The data showed that forensic population uses drugs to escape problems, to escape the grief of losing a child or loved one, using drugs as a means of "self-medicating," to "relax," or to relieve stress (see Table 1). Overall, this escape response was mentioned similarly between the two groups, amounting to a total of twenty-five times, the second most frequent response type for reasons to use drugs. Similarly, responses related to addiction, which included "addiction," "to get high," "desire" or "craving," "habit," and "like it," were cited twenty-two times between the two groups. Mentions of physical reasons and social reasons were less frequent, six and twelve times mentioned in total respectively.

Table 4

A Documented Experience of Chemical Impact of Alcohol and Street Drugs on the Mood and Behavior

Street drugs/alcohol	Impact of street drugs and alcohol
Alcohol	Drowsy, isolated, confident, friendly, happy, paranoid, memory loss, passing out, violent, and experience of dry mouth or out of saliva
Black beauty	Rage
Crack	Confuse, paranoid, loving, sexy, crazy, passive, living in isolation, thirsty and hungry
	And violent
Cocaine	Feeling good, paranoid, talkative, hallucinating, hungry, thirsty, and nervous
Crystal	Confident
Ecstasy	Crazy and sexy

Heroine	Rage, paranoid, imbalance
Marijuana	Feeling good, paranoid, confident
Methamphetamine	Alert, paranoid, feeling fine, rage, loving, talkative, drowsy, and euphoric, hair loss and mouth numb.
Pot	Crazy, confused, drowsy, imbalance, violent
Sham	Imbalance
Steroid	Feeling on top of the world and do not care about anything or feel fatigued or stressed

Feelings after Using Drugs

This area of drug and alcohol treatment should never be passed by unnoticed. Anticipated feeling management or AFM should be central in drug and alcohol treatment including trigger, cognition, and behavior. The reason people go shopping for street prescription drugs and alcohol is because they have an anticipated feeling to reach or attain if and when the drug or alcohol becomes available. Anticipated feelings and real feelings or effects must be identified and studied for the purpose of learning about the chemical nature of the drug, how people that have used it describe its impact overall and what that would have done to the person's overall physical health, organs, cognition, feelings, behavior, and other faculties of mental health identified and listed in this study. This is why from the data the author wanted to know how the impact has been described and documented in order to learn the difference between perceived or anticipated feelings, how they lead to the seeking and use of drugs as in Table 2, and the real reasons after the drug is ingested. This is important because people seek drugs or do drug shopping because they want to achieve a desired outcome or feeling. The key is finding out the difference between anticipated and real feelings before and after the drug is injected or after the addict self-medicates. Therefore, the second thematic category developed was from the descriptions of participants from the data of their feelings when using drugs and after they used. This chemical impact of different drugs' effect on the users is important to learn about the difference of the chemical effect of different drugs from the experiences of users. The data were categorized into five clusters of responses. These included: negative emotional response, physical symptoms, positive emotional response, self-perception, and social perception. Each is discussed.

Negative emotional response to using drugs included elements of feelings of depression, feeling unwanted or suicidal, low self-esteem, sadness, or the world being against you. In addition, this cluster included emotional responses of "anger," "aggression," "rage," or "violence," "panic" or "paranoia," "confusion," "shame" or "embarrassment," "guilt," "apathy," and the feeling of being "imbalanced." With eighteen mentions related to negative emotional responses, this represented the most common cluster of responses related to feelings when using drugs.

Physical symptoms were noted thirteen times between the groups. These elements included feelings of physical discomfort or illness. The specific responses given by participants included "dizziness," "sickness," "being hungry, thirsty, tired, drowsy," "having a poor appetite," "an increased sexual desire," and "feeling intoxicated."

Positive emotional responses were also noted by group participants in terms of their feelings when using drugs. These positive responses included feeling happy, "being on top of the world," "good," "confident," "peaceful," and "loving." It was noted that these positive emotional responses were mentioned a total of eight times, more than half as few as the negative emotional responses.

Feelings related to individual self-perception were also noted. These included feelings of being "crazy," "abnormal," "normal," "watchful" or "alert," and "different." These feelings were described by participants a total of seven times.

Feelings stemming from drug-use related to social perceptions were also described by participants. These included being "talkative," "friendly," and "sociable," to being "passive," "secretive," or "isolated," and "free." These descriptions grouped as social perceptions were noted a total of seven times as well. Regarding feeling and drug use, sometimes drugs that we think have good feelings may have some negative side effect on a person's mental, physical, social, and spiritual abilities. How do I know this? Well, the answer is simple: check what studies have been done that present both sides of a street drug before concluding it is all safe. What you consider safe in one area or relief may not be in other areas of the human dimension. Let me explain, from the USC Trojan, Winter, 2012, p. 6, which states, "Recreational marijuana use is linked to increased risk of testicular cancer, according to a new research from the Keck School of Medicine of USC. According to a leading scientist Victoria Cortessis, it is found that pot smokers were twice as likely to have testicular cancers of the non-seminoma subtype and mixed germ-cell tumors. Testicular cancer is most diagnosed in men aged from fifteen to forty-five years. Striking this balance is always important to get a good picture though you might disagree with the findings. Also, if there are negatives, what precautionary steps should both patients and clinicians take? What precautionary steps will you take with a client that is having a key to a car if that client is self-medicating on street drugs that cause ongoing drowsiness and sleepiness? These are questions you ask after a good analysis is completed.

Problems from Using Drugs

The third thematic category included the problems associated with the use of drugs. These perceived problems were grouped into five clusters of responses. These included responses related to emotional/psychological problems, physical/health problems, social problems, financial/legal problems, and academic/work problems.

Emotional or psychological problems were described by participants a total of forty-one times, representing the most common problems cited by participants. These responses were numerous and varied. Specific responses included obsession, paranoia, bad temper, anger, being argumentative, feeling guilt or shame, feeling misunderstood, feeling numb, depressed, or suicidal, feeling sad or nervous, violence, mental problems, delusional or having hallucinations, forgetfulness, perceived infallibility or recklessness, lack of confidence, feeling uneven or having a chemical imbalance, and feeling unsatisfied. The variety of responses is demonstrated and illustrates the psychological effects of drugs on each individual.

Physical or health problems were noted a total of thirty-seven times between the two groups. Responses under this cluster included changes in appearance, such as poor hygiene, body odor red eyes or black teeth; allergies; upset stomach or illness; sore bones; rashes; feeling uncomfortable; hunger; dependence; dry mouth; impaired sexual performance; blackouts; getting hurt or injured (e.g., getting shot);

not knowing what is in the drug or mixing drugs; relapse; abusing or overdosing; stress; insomnia or sleeping problems; poor appetite; and weakness. These represent the actual textual responses given by participants of physical problems associated with the use of drugs, and most often represent the participants' personal experiences.

Social problems occurred twenty-nine times. Responses included homelessness, lying, social isolation, social problems, doing things you are not supposed to do (e.g., stealing), tardiness, missing a normal life, sex crazed, peer pressure or trying to be popular, relationship problems, lack of cooperation, and unable to be oneself. Although these responses represent perceptions of the participants in terms of the problems associated with drug use, the similarity to the feelings and causes resulting from drug use are noted.

Another group of problems associated with drug use included financial and legal problems. These problems were specifically described as financial problems, legal problems, getting arrested, being jail, not paying bills, spending money on friends, dealing drugs, stealing from family or friends, pawning, and prostitution.

Finally, four instances of participants noting academic or work problems related to drug use were recorded in the data. These elements included missing school or work, quitting job, and academic problems. This cluster of responses was closely related to financial problems, although it was kept separate for the analysis. Overall, a diverse response pattern in terms of problems associated with drug use sheds light on the different experiences of the group participants, which can contribute to an understanding of the background for use and the understanding of particular triggers.

Causes for Relapse

The fourth thematic category revealed from the data analysis was related to the responses given with regard to why people relapse. There are personal reasons for relapse and/or perceptions of other reasons for relapse (Table 3). The responses also shed light on potential relapse triggers. Within this category are included social reasons, personal identification as an addict, emotional reasons, and environmental or community triggers of specific people, places, or things. Social reasons included family problems, lack of support system, social situations, and drop out of AA/NA, celebrating freedom, fun, and boredom. Personal identification as an addict included statements of self-identification ("the way we are" or "live their life with drugs"), self-proclaimed as "addicted," loss of willpower, and loss of responsibility/lack of priority. Emotional reasons were emotional problems ("anger," "resentment," or "sadness"), to feel better, death, and depression. Last but not the least, it is environmental or community factors or triggers such as people, places, or things that trigger the relapse. As you read through this section, it must be said there is always a difference between a person buying to use drugs and a person involved in the trade of selling drugs. The motivation and influence are different so are the triggers. I recalled visiting an individual just released from Detention Center in California. I was assigned to do the follow-up visit and monitor the drug court requirement of the individual and write a court report.

I recalled making an unannounced visit and found he was not following through with his AA requirement of three meetings a week. It was obvious he was using drugs again. I recalled discussing the noncompliance of the court order. I found the individual was selling drugs to support his wife and two children. He was not on any income. He mentioned finding a job that will hire a felon is a problem and worst meeting his family financial commitment now that he was home was building pressure to do anything to support his family. Also, it would take time to put in place a work program, making application for benefit, housing, etc. The individual mentioned that he got recruited to sell drugs, but in the process, he started using them again.

Table 5
Why People Relapse

	Group 1	Group 2	Total
Social reasons	**8**	**7**	**15**
Family problems	2	1	3
Lack of support system	1	1	2
Social situations	2	2	4
Drop out of AA/NA	1	1	2
Celebrate freedom	1	1	2

Fun	1		1
Boredom		1	1
Personal identification as addict and personal response	**6**	**7**	**13**
Self-identification: the way they live their life with drugs	2	1	3
Addicted	2	3	5
Lost the willpower	1	1	2
Loss of responsibility/lack of priorities	1	2	3
Emotional reasons	**4**	**8**	**12**
Emotional problems (anger, resentment, sadness)	2	4	6
To feel better	1	1	2
Death	1	1	2
Depression		2	2
Environment/community	**1**	**5**	**6**
Environment/triggers: people, places, things (including weed w/ meds, LSD w/food)	1	5	6

Personal Relapse Triggers

This served as the fifth and final thematic category for reconstructing the life and living of pretreatment relapse addiction. However, it was noted that responses to this category were limited to the second group only. As opposed to reasons for relapse, this category describes elements that participants felt to serve more specifically as triggers to relapse. Table 3 represents the responses in group two and the frequency of those responses. Key triggers, as noted, included social relationships and psychological elements, such as self-doubt or low self-esteem, anxiety or stress, grief, suicidal thoughts, or trying to be you. Social relationships served as the other commonly mentioned trigger. These elements included peer pressure or being around others who are still using drugs, personal relationships, maintaining a relationship with the drug dealer, and use during the holidays.

The ability to take these perceived personal triggers and direct therapy toward the most pressing triggers for the group is the value of the qualitative therapy method. The incidence of social triggers was to be expected from the literature reviewed; however, the prevalence of psychological factors is relevant, as these intrinsic factors can be addressed in therapy, whereas external triggers such as social relationships can be more difficult to address directly. In addition, the relatively low incidence of physical triggers was also noted.

Table 6
Personal Relapse Triggers

	Total
Social relationships	**8**
Peer pressure/others still using	3
Staff relationship	1
Abusive relationships	1
Personal relationships	1
Contact with drug dealer	1
Holiday use	1
Psychological	**7**
Self-doubt/low self-esteem	2
Stress/anxiety	2
Suicidal thoughts	1
Dealing with the loss of a friend	1
Being yourself	1
Financial problems	**4**

Not receiving benefit checks	1
Bills piling up	1
Loss of job	1
Not able to live comfortably	1
Physical	**2**
Desire/craving to get high	1
Going off meds	1

Summary of Results

For the information obtained from data, the qualitative approach was seen to obtain a comprehensive understanding of a small group or groups of individuals with drug addiction and mental health diagnoses. Results indicate social, psychological, financial, and physical relapse triggers as well as personal, social, environmental, and emotional perceived causes for relapse specific to the group or individuals. Specific perceived causes of relapse included social situations or social problems, personal identification as an addict, emotional problems (sadness, anger, aggression, depression), and environment/community triggers of specific people, places, and things. Personal relapse triggers were noted to vary according to the individual; however, social relationships, especially in terms of peer pressure with others still using drugs around you, and psychological factors of self-doubt, low self-esteem, stress, and anxiety were felt to serve as relapse triggers. This in-depth understanding of factors that can induce relapse can be used to more effectively reconstruct the pretreatment relapse life and living experience of individuals and also for constructing a clean and sober life and living for these individuals, their families and relatives. The qualitative group approach is therefore suggested as an effective means of obtaining, through therapeutic practice, critical understanding of relapse triggers in order to promote a more relevant, personalized, and successful treatment plan for the prevention of relapse. Also, a clinician treating a patient or client will use this information not only to reconstruct but also to construct a clean and sober life envisioned by the client. A clinician may also address other issues of concern with the construction treatment planning phase, including, but not limited to safety, relapse prevention training and skills, medication, mental health, social, spiritual, and physical health. But therapies and clinicians can go so far in responding to the chemical effect of drugs and alcohol. Community involvement is definitely required including drugs and alcohol producers (legalize producers) to do what is possible to eliminate the known chemical risk in their products before it is made available to the public.

CONCLUSIONS

In this final analysis, the author compiled into a report the information about understanding pretreatment relapse triggers and what driving demand for drug use among forensic individuals is. In addition, a theory was generated that was grounded in the information extracted from the data to explain why forensic mentally ill individuals relapse. The results and generated theory provide the conclusions of the study.

Review of the Findings

A review of the findings is presented according to the research questions of the study.

Analysis Question 1: According to the data, what will the data tell the author/research about the nature of addiction trigger?

The results of the study from the data analysis demonstrate the multilevel effects of personal experience on personal relapse. External and internal factors were found and described by participants from the community and family level to an individual level. Relapse triggers were described by participants in terms of social and environmental factors, which, from the review of the literature, was somewhat expected. However, participants also noted individual, intrinsic factors, such as emotional states or problems that served to precipitate relapse, such as depression, sadness, aggression, anger, stress/anxiety, low self-esteem, and self-doubt. The study suggests the critical nature of addressing these psychological responses to drug use not only as a COD but also as a specific trigger for relapse.

Analysis Question 2: What are the causes, patterns, and categories of pretreatment addiction relapse triggers experienced by forensic individuals found in the data proposed for analysis?

According to the findings revealed from the data analysis, participants revealed a variety of causes for addiction relapse. The most common causes given by these group participants included social situations and social problems such as family problems and daily social situations and social relationships, including environmental triggers within the community of people, places, and things that call to mind using behaviors (peer pressure, or being around others who are still using); emotional problems such as anger, aggression, extreme sadness, or depression; and behaviors associated with a personal identification as an addict. Personal psychological triggers associated with self-doubt, low self-esteem, and stress and/or anxiety were also reported by participants often.

These perceptions also shed light on the nature of relapse specifically for this population. Although what would be considered to be typical relapse triggers according to the research, such as social situations/relationships, environmental, and community triggers, this population with COD also noted psychological factors of emotional problems, self-doubt, anxiety, and personal identification as an addict as additional or compounding addiction triggers.

Analysis Question 3: Based on the study, what is the most effective way of treating pretreatment addiction relapse triggers?

According to the findings revealed in this study, providing assistance in developing strategies to handle social situations, relationships, and problems without relapsing would be beneficial to reducing the rate of relapse. Through the qualitative group approach, these strategies can be developed for very specific circumstances; for example, one participant noted a common trigger of food, due to the previous habit of taking LSD with food. A specific strategy can be developed for this individual in terms of finding an appropriate action plan for dealing with that specific trigger. Other triggers are more general and can incorporate the use of a more general, group-designed strategy, such as maintaining a support group to deal with social or emotional support issues that may arise.

It is noted, however, that within this population of individuals with COD, specific attention should be given to emotional/psychological responses to drug use and/or relapse. Counseling directed toward treatment processes for depression, mood disorders, general anxiety, or stress management, as well as issues of self-doubt and self-esteem, need to be added as a relapse prevention strategy. The personal identification of these individuals with drug use should also be addressed, perhaps through a focus on a reexamination of the individual and their personal strengths and weaknesses to develop a more concrete perception of self outside the realm of drug use.

Analysis Question 4: How does the qualitative group therapy process for ERA, which targets the revealed risks and relapse triggers contribute to current research understanding of pretreatment addiction relapse triggers and prompt recommendation for relapse prevention and discharge readiness before a client is released or discharged into the same or similar community he or she was arrested from?

The author discovered he could adapt qualitative research methodology into a group therapy process for understanding pretreatment addiction relapse triggers. The author looked at many other therapy models and research models and decided on qualitative method as the viable possibility with good potential for identifying and understanding pretreatment addiction in a large group of over thirty individuals. The approach was successful at determining the varied relapse factors for individuals as well as more common relapse responses given by the group. As such, the approach can be used by clinicians facilitating such education, to provide a greater level of knowledge and understanding of the individual factors representing real risks for these group participants that need to be addressed for successful relapse prevention. Without addressing the predominant relapse triggers for these individuals, it becomes more likely that the relapse prevention will fail to be effective.

Results from this study also underscore the importance of simultaneous treatment of the underlying co-occurring disorders and the reported psychological effects of drug use within this population, as psychological problems were noted not only as a cause for initial drug use and relapse but also as a personal trigger for these participants.

Discussion and Treatment

Group Therapy Approach

The result from the data analysis underscores how important it is to use the qualitative therapy approach when processing drug and alcohol group because of the potential it offers in data information. Also, the importance of analytic data process and the result we see from this study could not be overstated as the right direction to go in drug and alcohol treatment. The future drug treatment from now on will require both the approaches for identifying, categorizing, developing patterns and risk levels of pretreatment addiction relapse trigger, or any other trigger similar approach may be used. What this means is that the clinician will have a therapy model designed for drug and alcohol and analysis steps for analyzing relapse trigger. The potential is limitless as to where this science goes from this study and the new tools that will make it possible to scan a data; a software can do all the work in terms of analysis, identification, categorizing, patterns, and identify trigger risk levels for treatment planning. Also, the benefit is immense, and gone are the days when we talk about triggers but are unable to identify them, categorize them, develop patterns, show what triggers you have identified and the risk levels. The clinical potential is also immense because you can back your drug and alcohol billing and treatment intervention with scientific analysis. I am certain when we think of the possibilities this single study has unfolded and where we go from here in forensic addiction treatment. This is not added work to a therapist but a new opportunity to enhance treatment and billing practice and also for potential to specialize in qualitative therapy practice and data analysis. Data analysis shows many things about addiction disease. Some we may have known, but the rest is new. But what is important from now on is that we know the reason, reasons, or variables contributing to the demand for drug use and ongoing use and relapse in the Inland Empire. This should help us understand the plight of a friend or a member of your family or patient you have seen battling with drug, alcohol, and prescription drug shopping and cannot get over or stop using and relapsing. It will take time to stop as you wish because they are experiencing many triggers in the environment contributing to their relapse behavior. But you and I can help. How we use this knowledge to develop treatment or a plan-effective response will be the next step.

A clinician contemplating using qualitative method and analysis in group treatment can incorporate the Mall group approach foci of hospitalization to complete the treatment plan for clients and individual. *The Mall* is a name for a centralized approach to the delivery of psycho education. The Mall provides an opportunity for individuals and staff to come together to participate in services. The Mall represents a centralized system of programs, rather than a reference to a specific building or certain location (Patton State Hospital, 2007). Each Mall is assigned a clinician to provide therapeutic and rehabilitation services to individuals or groups. The Mall is divided into five functional malls, each running up to eleven recovery clinics, based on the following foci of hospitalization (Patton State Hospital, 2007). There is no ninth focus.

Focus 1	Psychiatric, psychological, or mental state
Focus 2	Social skills and self-esteem
Focus 3	Dangerous impulsivity and anger problems
Focus 4	Hope and spirituality
Focus 5	Substance abuse
Focus 6	Medical, health, and wellness states

Focus 7   Incompetence to stand trial
Focus 8   School and education
Focus 10   Stress, leisure, and recreation
Focus 11   Discharge readiness, community integration, job
              training, education, and social support

Relating these results to prior research in chapter two enables us to decipher the results in terms of practice. Relapse is not a sudden event, but rather the culmination of a chain of events and behaviors. Triggers and stressors are frequently highly individualized (Kelly et al., 2007). Therefore, in the prevention of relapse, it is important to consider individual triggers and stressors in order to assist the individual to learn to prevent or minimize their own relapse risk (Kelly et al., 2007).

The results from this study demonstrate causes and specific relapse triggers that both align with previous research and shed light on new concepts. Common triggers previously identified in the literature review were also found in the data used in the analyses and are consistent with stressors. Carroll (1998) described common triggers of being around people with whom one previously used drugs: having money, getting paid, drinking, being involved in a social situation, and experiencing certain affective states such as anxiety, depression, or joy. A comparative study of the triggers in the analysis was also compared with many common triggers in the literature review. These triggers include social situations and social problems such as family problems and daily social situations and social relationships, including abusive relationships, lack of support, boredom, holidays, peer pressure, being around others who are using or with whom the individual used drugs prior to treatment, or other situations or people that call to mind using behaviors; emotional problems such as anger, aggression, extreme sadness, anxiety, stress, or depression.

Many of these elements were also noted by NIDA (2009), such as family and friends, socio-community status, peer pressure, physical and sexual abuse, stress, parental involvement, and the critical developmental stages in a person's life that will cause or predispose a person to be vulnerable to drug use. The results also align with evidence that family problems and poverty are also possible triggers for drug and alcohol use (Costello et al., 2006; Rosenbloom, 2009).

In addition to these relapse triggers identified in previous research in the literature review, information from participants in the data described specific behaviors associated with a personal identification as an addict and personal psychological triggers associated with depression, suicidal thoughts, self-doubt, low self-esteem, and grief. Self-identification as an addict was described in terms of "it's the way I am" or that they "live their life with drugs." Some participants simply labeled themselves as an addict, which they described as a reason to relapse. Others described a loss of willpower or loss of responsibility or lack of priority associated with self-identification as an addict. Noted to a lesser degree were financial and academic or work problems serving as stressors and promoting relapse.

Turning more specifically to the population with COD, drug or alcohol use has been shown to increase psychiatric problems, particularly among young people, of individuals suffering from depression, anxiety, and antisocial personality disorders (Califano, 2006). Given this claim, if these psychiatric disorders also serve as relapse triggers, as suggested by participants in this study, effective identification and treatment becomes critical to their success. According to the review of the literature, clinicians have not been able to gather an adequate understanding of relapse triggers and experiences, an understanding of why forensic mentally ill individuals relapse as they do, or an understanding of the impact of substances, which is necessary for planning relapse intervention. These results provide insight into the specific factors perceived by a population of forensic mentally ill individuals to trigger a relapse.

Prior research using qualitative measures has been used to explore relapse prevention and/or drug use. The findings from a study by Smith (2006) provided participant suggestions for the use of interpersonal reflection as well as cognitive and action-based coping skills as a means of avoiding relapse. Research by Harris et al. (2005) identified not only obstacles to recovery that align with this current research, such as battles with depression and despair, destructive habits and patterns, and lack of personal control, but also supportive factors of connection, self-awareness, a sense of purpose and meaning, and spirituality that can be used as additional information to incorporate into treatment.

Results of this study confirm the position of the Center for Substance Abuse Treatment (CSAT, 2005, 2007) in which positive treatment results for individuals with co-occurring disorders (COD) such as mental illness and substance abuse are best achieved through addressing both the substance abuse and the mental illness within a shared context, supporting the need for targeted treatment for the prevention of relapse. However, without specific details and understanding of precise individual triggers, as are provided through the qualitative group therapy approach, those dealing simultaneously with mental illness and substance abuse may represent the poor treatment outcomes that have been reported for this cohort to date (CSAT, 2005, 2007).

The therapist, clinician, or treatment program will have to tune to the environment to learn about the triggers in the environment and also pay attention to issues in the environment that may impact their client behavior. They may then use that information to reconstruct the client's or individual's life before a relapse occurred. A clinician will have to judge the ideal environment for client sobriety in a neighborhood where triggers for relapse are high, restriction on employment for felons and socioeconomic challenges are very high, making living conditions and earning difficulty. Also, a subject of focus will include the following but not limited to old friends, easy access to drugs, alcohol and shopping for prescription drugs, paraphernalia and places or hideouts that help facilitate secrecy and relapse behavior. Also, some clients may not be ready to deal with family relationship upon release or know what to do in case their sobriety is threatened. It is important from this analysis to use qualitative therapy developed for trigger exploration, process, and identification in group therapy. Also, important is to analyze the pretreatment relapse triggers for understanding categories, patterns and risk an individual or group may have been exposed to or will be if released to the same or similar community where they used drugs, relapsed, and were arrested from. Why? It is because triggers are a harsh reality, one that is rarely analyzed using scientific method. It is no excuse now that we have a qualitative therapy model and the analysis steps in place to get the job done for enhancing drug and alcohol therapy and minimize relapse prevention alongside cognitive behavior therapy. A clinician will have to go beyond cognitive and behavior modification to identify and work with specific triggers in the client's environment or community. Alcohol treatment should not be confined in therapy groups, office, or consultation therapy room. Working with the person and triggers will include both office and community or family.

Conclusion

The future of drug and alcohol will not be the same as data analysis is taking center stage in health care not only for billing but also in this case for study and analysis of addiction treatment. Analysis will help us understand vectors and triggers in any disease, including addiction. This is why it is important now that we have a therapy model discovered and developed for working with drug and alcohol population to start positioning students and therapists to train on qualitative therapy skills and analysis techniques.

Drug treatment should include showing trigger analysis in real time and sharing the information with the patients and parties involved. This is not an extra burden beyond doing groups or individual therapy but a step in the right direction to show that triggers are real and are contributing to relapse behavior. You cannot change the mind, thoughts, feelings, and addictive behavior if you fail to identify the relapse triggers involved in contributing to the relapse behavior and show how you will address each relevant trigger overall in developing relapse prevention goals and objectives. Running groups and individual therapy is different from data study and analysis as you have seen demonstrated in this study. Trigger identification and analysis will be a specialized profession that will contribute not only to billing but also to drug and alcohol treatment development in the twenty-first century.

As a therapist, you should never forget that there are millions of individuals hooked on to drugs and alcohol night and day, making stops on the way home in liquor stores and corners for street drugs. Addicts are not only battling with drugs and relapse behavior but also with triggers, and these must be addressed in therapy. Also, addiction comes with a lost identity that does not reflect the true person's self-worth. Self-worth and identity is what you are born with not what your behavior is and the chemical addiction problem you are stuck with. Addiction treatment should address an individual's identity as the image and likeness of a divine being, which has been undermined due to being in chemical addiction and the behavior exhibited thereby. We are only allowed to be one thing, and that is what we are: the image and likeness of God, and any other thing you have become is not you but a lost identity you must reclaim in recovery. Recovery is like going to recover what is left from a burnt house. What are you addicted to? There are a lot of things that you easily become addicted to, but however desirable they are, you must try to identify and analyze the triggers that got you addicted.

Summary

The author hopes that by now he has provided answers to the four questions developed for this research in chapter one. The proposal to analyze data for the answers has been met with. It is hoped the author has contributed to the field of addiction psychology by describing the use of scientific analysis in explaining as to what else beyond mental status and behavior is driving individuals to use drugs. The use of qualitative therapy and qualitative analysis steps and software is just the beginning of pretreatment addiction relapse triggers often associated with relapse behavior. In case you have been wondering trying to understand why some folks or relatives or persons you know have not stopped using drugs, the author hopes he has provided the information that should guide treatment intervention. The author has also learned in the process the hidden phenomena of drug and alcohol use.

According to Young et al. (2001), in the general population, the rate of recidivism is 86% two years after treatment, with the majority of the relapses occurring within six months of treatment. The author in the previous chapter analyzed factors driving demand for drug use among forensic population in the United States. Now that we know the answers, how is that different from the metaphysical cause in the temptation of Jesus and the general psychology explanation for what is driving human demand for drug use and what treatment option is best and applicable?

Studies have shown limited treatment success for substance abusers. This book offers hope that therapists could improve their group treatment and discharge relapse prevention intervention with improved knowledge and understanding of pretreatment triggers for reconstructing and constructing drug treatment using a qualitative model and approach.

Now that we have the analysis report, our next step is thinking about what are the appropriate treatment goals and objectives? It is good to start the discussion on treatment by reviewing what the options and responses are. Therefore, the author has included what the ideas are as follows:

1. Liberalize drug use and prevent drug cartel from making profits. Some suggested that liberalizing drug use will result in federal tax income or local state tax income increase.
2. Other suggestion calls for medical allowance only in the case of individuals in pain or those who are terminally ill.
3. Law enforcement response raid, arrest, convict and jail time or divergent programs including drug court treatment.
4. Clinicians recommend psycho-educational group with use of psychotherapy possibly cognitive behavior therapy (CBT) for treatment.
5. Psychologists recommend treatment that will include test and behavior modification and reward approach.
6. Psychiatrists recommend drug and alcohol detox including inpatient treatment plus psychiatric treatment if there are signs of drug use and psychiatric problems like depression or person hears voices or sees things and outpatient treatment upon discharge including random drug test, unexpected home visits, attend three AA/NA a week and showing up in court when on calendar.
7. Probation registration, visits, and also notifying the probation officer of any change of address.

But treatment approach or recommendation or policy will have to be consistent with analysis of specific pretreatment relapse triggers than general triggers. Whatever recommendation is reached, it must seek to minimize triggers and relapse or the driving demand for drug use.

Most of the familiar treatment approaches have been centered on stopping the use of obtaining drug and alcohol, cognitive behavior modification, and very recently combination of mental health treatment, a subject which was always kept separate until it was clear that individuals with chemical addiction may also have mental challenges. What has not been included in the treatment package is what the discovery of qualitative therapy has uncovered, which is pretreatment relapse triggers as environmental and social issues for reconstructing pretreatment relapse life for constructing a clean and sober life with other aspects of care that are consistent with the four-dimensional structures of a person's life: physical, mental, social, and spiritual.

Also, another key aspect often overlooked by a clinician is the fact that majority of individuals in forensic treatment come to treatment after they are arrested for drug and alcohol use or other related crimes against a person, property, or health hazard behavior, including the sale and distribution of street drugs. Drug treatment must not only focus on drug use, cognitive issues, mental health and behavior challenges, but treatment must also attempt to address the illegality of the demand and behavior of drug use, an approach generally overlooked in treatment. Individuals can benefit a lot if they are allowed to process criminal thinking and behaviors alongside mental health, drug and alcohol problems. Why is this important? It is important because individuals that come to treatment come after they have been arrested and then are sent for treatment. Therefore, addressing the issue of arrest and criminal behavior through use of knowledge of the law in group process is highly warranted. As a therapist, I remember starting a group called "Criminal Thinking and Law." In this group, I was able to also use my legal knowledge to address some of the key issues of law related to criminal behavior and why an individual should ask before initiating a behavior if it is legal. Is it allowed by law, or will it result in crime against a person, property, or health problems? From experience, a lot of the individuals do not process behavior with a legal mind; they act out of pressure from people, places, and things or out of instinct.

Therefore, from forensic treatment experience, effective treatment of alcohol and street drugs will include treatment aimed at assessing the environment for pretreatment relapse triggers, working on the feelings and legal awareness of behavior.

In this book, you have seen how qualitative group therapy or Q therapy is a valuable tool for identifying pretreatment relapse triggers for reconstructing and constructing treatment. Q therapy is also an effective tool for identifying and understanding pretreatment relapse triggers for cognitive behavior therapy practice. It is useful for understanding feelings before and after reaction to particular street drugs or alcohol use. The chemical effect of street drugs on users is essential for treatment. Managing how an addict expects to feel before he or she uses a specific drug or combination is important for relapse prevention. Addiction treatment must not only be focused on cognitive and behavior modification but also take a hard look at the individual's feelings. Why is this important? We have included the impact and effect of drugs or combination of drugs in the analysis because the author for experience thinks it is important to process the experience of what an individual or group wants to feel and how they felt after they ingested or self-administered the drug. Sometimes expected feelings are different from perceived or real feelings. It is important you work on feelings and suggest what else is available other than chemicals to improve feelings. We are creatures that always want to experience something or numb our feelings to escape some unpleasant situation or problem. It is also important to learn how much harm overexposure to chemical substances has caused to a person's health, system, or internal organs. Looks or performance are not the best indicators that a person's system or organs are working; we expect that is the case, but my experience has taught me it is not always the case. Health is based on many things, including the physical system and all organs working well. You do not want a client you are treating to drop dead from a heart attack or kidney failure when you did not request a referral for a system or organ checks. You have a responsibility to ensure the safety of a client once in your care, and part of the safety is in addressing health issues if you know the individual has been using drugs for very long time and has a history or pattern of drug abuse and overdose.

There is always a reason why drug users want to avoid being mentally alert and also change or alter their feelings. Therefore, processing this issue with a client or individual is important for assessing whether or not the initial before purchasing and using the drug is any different from the real effect after the drug is used or self-administered. A counselor who reported his client was using two drugs at a time was asked what the difference is. Why is this important to know? From experience, some people use street drugs for different reasons and expectations including but not limited to avoiding stage fright that comes from all eyes on them while performing on stage, to numb their shy feelings when socializing, escape social problems, cope with hardship and crisis, and escape pain or want to experience Christmas or have a happy feeling every day. They may also want to avoid situations including holidays that have sad memories. Individuals with any of these expectations may sabotage any plans to stay clean and sober. But if they are not getting the desired results, they may be willing to look for alternatives and cooperate with the therapist. Also, some drugs are capable of having negative and positive effects at the same time. Alcohol may help a user feel confident before a group or loosen up to interact after it is self-administered, but it also has a negative or downside effect. Alcohol can also cause dry mouth or make a person slow down because it affects the central nervous system or CNS. These kinds of contrasts can be monitored by family members or the individuals for process purposes and relapse awareness.

The main interest now that the book is published is to see how qualitative therapy and qualitative analysis lead the way in drug and alcohol pretreatment addiction relapse trigger for identifying, processing, and analyzing categories, patterns, and trigger risk level not only for billing purpose but also for understanding relapse triggers and developing appropriate treatment goals and objectives, also how the information will be utilized for training purpose in addiction trigger data analysis and development of treatment programs. The research has paved the way for interest in this field of data analysis as seen taking roots in other health services. Data analysis offers a great potential for study and analysis for understanding vectors and triggers. With this understanding, we learn that addiction is not only a mental, cognitive, and behavioral problem, but a trigger issue as well and what are we doing working with addicts with complex social and environmental unresolved triggers recurring now and then triggering relapse. Is our drug treatment ready to deal with environmental triggers or just the person? And how do we go about that to prevent ongoing and repeated relapse or recidivism? This is why this book was written to lead the way on issues that should concern every therapist and what we should be doing in responding to addiction diseases.

Finally, as an author, my personal commitment now is to use this information on pretreatment relapse triggers as reference material to raise awareness about pretreatment addiction relapse triggers, qualitative therapy potential, and analysis for understanding pretreatment addiction triggers so that clinicians, psychologists, clinical social workers, families, law enforcement agencies, drug courts, policy makers, program managers, students, colleges, and universities can be aware of pretreatment triggers in communities that contribute or will continue to contribute to drug use and relapse and do something about it. Also, I will like to continue to teach how to use and apply qualitative or Q therapy in groups and the benefit it offers for identifying pretreatment relapse triggers. It is expected that qualitative therapy and data analysis in drug and alcohol treatment will grow because of its treatment benefits for understanding pretreatment addiction relapse trigger and its risk level to patients or individuals for planning treatment goals and objectives.

REFERENCES

American Psychiatric Association. (2004). *Diagnostic and statistical manual of mental disorders* (4th ed.). Washington, DC: Author.

Beck, A. (1993). *Cognitive therapy and the emotional disorders.* New York, NY: Penguin.

Beck, J. S. (1995). *Cognitive therapy.* New York, NY: Guildford press.

Boggan, W. (2008). *Alcohol and you.* Retrieved from http://www.chemcase.com/alcohol

Bradizza, C. M., & Stasiewicz, P. R. (2003). Qualitative analysis of high-risk drug and alcohol-use situations among severely mentally ill substance abusers. *Journal of Addictive Behavior, 28,* 157-69. Retrieved from http://www.sciencedirect.com

Braun, V., & Clarke, V. (2006). Using thematic analysis in psychology. *Qualitative Research in Psychology, 3*(2), 77-101. doi: 10.1191/1478088706qp063oa

Califano, J. A. (2006). Alcohol and teen drinking. *National Center on Addiction and Substance Abuse.* Retrieved from http://www.focusas.com/Alcohol.html

California Department of Alcohol and Drug Programs. (2010). *Dual diagnosis and co-occurring disorders history.* Retrieved from http://www.adp.ca.gov/COD/history.shtml

California Department of Alcohol and Drug Programs Co-Occurring Disorders Unit. (2010). *Co-occurring program planning guide for early intervention under the Mental Health Services Act (MHSA).* Retrieved from http://www.adp.ca.gov/COD/pdf/PEI_Guide.pdf

California Department of Mental Health, State Hospital. (2007). *Administrative directive # 1.00.* Retrieved from Patton State Hospital Intranet.

Carroll, M. (1998). *Therapy manual for drug addiction: A cognitive behavior approach.* US Department of Health and Human Services. Retrieved from http://www.encyclopedia.com/topic/cognition_behavior_therapy.aspx

Center for Substance Abuse Treatment. (2005). *Substance abuse treatment for persons with co-occurring disorders.* Treatment Improvement Protocol (TIP) Series 42. DHHS Publication No. (SMA) 05-3992. Rockville, MD: Substance Abuse and Mental Health Services Administration.

Center for Substance Abuse Treatment. (2007). *Screening, assessment, and treatment planning for persons with co-occurring disorders.* COCE Overview Paper 2. DHHS Publication No. (SMA) 07-4164. Rockville, MD: Substance Abuse and Mental Health Services Administration, and Center for Mental Health Services. Retrieved from http://www.coce.samhsa.gov/cod_resources/PDF/OP2-ScreeningandAssessment-8-13-07.pdf

Chenail, R. J., & Maione, P. (2009). *Sense-making in clinical qualitative research.* Retrieved from http://www.nova.edu/ssss/QR/QR3-1/sense.html

Cherry, K. (n.d.). *What is the amygdala?* Retrieved from http://psychology.about.com/od/aindex/g/amygdala.html

Costello, E. J., Sung, M., Worthman, C., & Angold, A. (2006). *Pubertal maturation and the development of alcohol use and abuse.* Retrieved from http://www.elsevier.com

---

Creswell, J. W. (2005). *Educational research: Planning, conducting, and evaluating quantitative and qualitative research*. Upper Saddle River, NJ: Pearson Education.

Creswell, J. W. (2005). *Educational research: Planning, conducting, and evaluating quantitative and qualitative research* (2nd ed.). Upper Saddle River, NJ: Pearson Education.

Creswell, J. W. (2007). *Educational research: Planning, conducting, and evaluating quantitative and qualitative research*. Upper Saddle River, NJ: Pearson Education.

Dean, D. A. (2009). *Drug addiction*. Retrieved from http://www.csun.edu/~vcpsyooh/students/drugs.html

Drug Addiction Triggers. (2010). Retrieved from http://www.tarzana.org

Drug-Rehabs.org. (2009). *Drug rehab and alcohol addiction treatment information*. Retrieved from http://www.drug-rehabs.org

Enkel, T., Spanagel, R., Vollmayr, B., & Schneider, M. (2010). Stress triggers anhedonia in rats bred for learned helplessness. *Behavioural Brain Research, 209*(1), 183-86. doi: 10.1016/j.bbr.2010.01.042

Everitt, B. J., & Robbins, T. W. (2005). Neural systems of reinforcement for drug addiction: From actions to habit to compulsion. *Nature Neuroscience, 8*(11), 1481-89. doi: 10.1038/nn1579

Glaser, B. G., & Strauss, A. L. (2009). *The discovery of grounded theory: Strategies for qualitative research* (4th ed.). New York, NY: Aldine Publishing Company.

Gonzales, A. R. (2005, April). Residential substance abuse treatment for state prisoners. *Bureau of Justice Assessment*. Washington, DC: US Office of Justice.

Harris, M., Fallot, R. D., & Berley, R. W. (2005). Special section on relapse prevention: Qualitative interviews on substance abuse relapse and prevention among female trauma survivors. *Psychiatric Services, 56,* 1292-96.

Hoepfl, M. C. (1997). *Choosing qualitative research: A primer for teaching education.* Retrieved from http://scholar.lib.vt.edu/journal/jee/v.html

Hunter, K., Hari, S., Egbu, C., & Kelly, J. (2005). Grounded theory: Its diversification and application through two examples from research studies on knowledge and value management. *Electronic Journal of Business Research Methods, 3*(1), 57-68.

Jaffe, A. (2010). *Trigger.* Retrieved from http://www.psychologytoday.com/blog/all_about_addiction/201003/triggers_and_relapse_craving_connection

Kelly, T. J., Gaither, J. M., & King, L. J. (2007). Relapse. In J. E. Lessenger & G. F. Roper (Eds.), *Drug courts: A new approach to treatment and rehabilitation* (pp. 377-88). New York, NY: Springer.

Krippendorff, K. (2004). *Content analysis: An introduction to its methodology.* Thousand Oaks, CA: Sage Publications.

Lombardo, T. (2005). *Behavior modification.* Thousand Oaks, CA: Sage Journals.

Le Doux, J. E. (2008). Amygdala. In *Scholarpedia.* Retrieved from http://www.scholarpedia.org/article/Amygdala2008

Leedy, P. D., & Ormrod, J. E. (2005). *Practical research* (8th ed.). Columbus, OH: Pearson Merrill Prentice Hall.

Luna, C. (2007). *Department of Mental Health, state hospital administrative directive #1,* 1-14.

Madigan, L. (2010). *Strategies for fighting meth.* Retrieved from http://www.illinoisattorneygeneral.gov/methnet/fightmeth/treatment.html

Mathison, C., Alexander, J., & Rizzo, J. (n.d.). *Introduction to the brain*. Retrieved from http://its.sdsu.edu/multimedia/mathison/limbic/index.html

Miller, W. R., & Rollnick, S. (2009) Ten things that motivational interviewing is not. *Behavioural and Cognitive Psychotherapy, 37,* 129-40.

Moustakas, C. E. (1994). *Phenomenological research methods.* Thousand Oaks, CA: Sage Publications.

National Institute on Drug Abuse. (2007). *Drugs, brains, and behavior: The science of addiction.* Retrieved from http://www.drugabuse.gov/tib/soa.html

National Institute on Drug Abuse. (2010). *Treatment recovery.* Retrieved from http://www.nida.nih.gov

Neill, J. (2009). *Analysis of professional literature: Class 6: Qualitative research I.* Retrieved from http://www.wilderdom.com/OEcourses/PROFLIT/Class6Qualitative1.htm

Neuendorf, K. A. (2002). *The content analysis guidebook.* Thousand Oaks, CA: Sage Publications.

Neuman, W. L. (2003). *Social research methods: Qualitative and quantitative approaches* (5th ed.). Boston, MA: Allyn & Bacon.

Office of National Drug Community Policy Executive office of the President. (2010). *Consequences of illicit drug use in America. Retrieved from* http://www.whitehouse.gov/sites/default/files/ondcp/Fact_Sheets/consequences_of_illicit_drug_use.pdf

Pate, L. (2009). *Triggers.* Retrieved from http://www.kci.org/meth_info/lori/triggers.htm

Patton, M. Q. (2002). *Qualitative research and evaluation methods.* Thousand Oaks, CA: Sage Publications.

Patton State Hospital. (2007, June 1). *Administrative directive, written plan for professional services # 1*, 1-4.

Polkinghorne, D. E. (2005). Language and meaning: Data collection in qualitative research. *Journal of Counseling Psychology, 52*(2), 137-45.

Rajasekaram, K., Kumar, J. R., & Venkatachalam, K. (2003). Increased neuronal nitric oxide synthase (nNOS) activity triggers picrotoxin-induced seizures in rats and evidence for participation of nNOS mechanism in the action of antiepileptic drugs. *Brain Research, 979*, 85-99. doi:10.1016/S0006-8993(03)02878-6

Ratcliff, D. (n.d.). *The qualitative research web page.* Retrieved from http://qualitative research.ratcliff.net

Reusch, W. (n.d.). Alcohols. *VirtualText of organic chemistry.* Retrieved from http://www.cem.msu.edu/~reusch/VirtualText/alcohol1.htm#alcnom

Rosenbloom, D. L. (2009). Holiday, triggers, and willpower. *Journal of Substance Abuse Treatment, 36*, 7.

Smith, C. H. S. (2006). *Exploring chronic sorrow as a relapse trigger in female victims of child abuse currently seeking treatment for substance abuse.* Doctoral dissertation, University of Arkansas for Medical Sciences. Retrieved from ProQuest database.

Sterk-Elifson, C. (1995). *Determining drug use patterns among women: The value of qualitative research methods.* Bethesda, MD: US Department of Health and Human Services, National Institute on Drug Abuse. Retrieved from PsycETRA. EBSCOhost

Tevyaw, T. O., Borsari, B., Colby, S. M., & Monti, P. M. (2007). Peer enhancement of a brief motivation intervention with mandated college students. *Psychology of Addictive Behaviors, 21*(1), 114-19. Retrieved from http://web.ebscohost.com/ehost/detail?Vid

Triggers. (2010). Retrieved from http://www.drug-rehabs.org/articles/114?

Urell, B. (2010). *Drug and Alcohol Addiction Relapse Triggers—A Really Simple Guide to Addiction Relapse Prevention.* Retrieved from http://ezinearticles.com/?Drug-and-Alcohol-Addiction-Relapse-Triggers—A-Really-Simple-Guide-to-Addiction-Relapse-Prevention&id=2088664

US Department of Health and Human Services (USHHS). (2009). *Substance abuse and Mental Health Services Administration Center for Substance Abuse Treatment.* Bethesda, MD: NIDA.

Vieten, C., Astin, J. A., Buscemi, R., & Galloway, G. P. (2010). Development of an acceptance-based coping intervention for alcohol dependence relapse prevention. *Substance Abuse, 31*(2), 108-16.

Wechsler, H., Dowdall, G., Maenner, G., Gledhill-Hoyt, J., & Lee, H. (1998). Changes in binge drinking and related problems among American college students between 1993 and 1997. *Journal of American College Health, 47*(2), 57-68.

Yin, R. K. (1994). *Case study research, design and methods.* Thousand Oaks, CA: Sage Publications.

Yoshikawa, H., Weisner, T. S., Kalil, A., & Way, N. (2008). Mixing qualitative and quantitative research in developmental science: Uses and methodological choices. *Developmental Psychology, 44*(2), 344-54. doi: 10.1037/0012-1649.44.2.344

Young, R. S., Joe, J. R, Hassin, J., & St. Clair, D. (2001). Addressing psychosocial issues and problems of co-morbidity for Native American clients with substance abuse problems: A conference proceedings. *American Indian and Alaska Native Mental Health Research, 10*, 2. Retrieved from ProQuest Psychological Journals.